T0230521

Clinician's Guide to Mycosis Fungoides

Pooya Khan Mohammad Beigi

Clinician's Guide
to Mycosis Fungoides

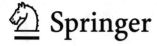 Springer

Pooya Khan Mohammad Beigi
Department of Health Management
New York Medical College
Valhalla, New York, USA

University of British Columbia
Vancouver, British Columbia, Canada

Misdiagnosis Association
Seattle, Washington, USA

ISBN 978-3-319-83854-0   ISBN 978-3-319-47907-1   (eBook)
DOI 10.1007/978-3-319-47907-1

Printed on acid-free paper

This Springer imprint is published by Springer Nature
The registered company is Springer International Publishing AG
The registered company address is: Gewerbestrasse 11, 6330 Cham, Switzerland

To a real hero
Mohammad Khan Mohammad Beigi
who inspired me to achieve and succeed
by focusing only ever on the goal
and never on the obstacles

and

To a real teacher
Parvin Mojabi
to whom I owe my life and all
that I have accomplished and become

and

To a real princess
Sherry Jalalian
who unceasingly encouraged me
with her patience, without which I would
not have been able to persevere
in spite of my humanity

Foreword

In this textbook, Dr. Pooya Khan Mohammad Beigi and collaborators provide a comprehensive summary of the state of the management of the most common cutaneous T-cell lymphomas (CTCL): mycosis fungoides/Sézary syndrome. They succinctly address the history, etiology, and management of this challenging disease.

We are still in an era where there is no clear algorithm for the management of this disease, and consequently, this brief and precise summation of our knowledge is both timely and easy to digest. I am sure anyone who is involved in the management of CTCL will find this enjoyable reading, whether that be an introduction to this disease or refresher for the experienced clinician.

There are less than a handful of randomized trials in CTCL, and so I am sure the reader will find the author's investigation into the use of PUVA+/− interferon highlights many issues we face in managing the patient with this disease.

We are entering an era of molecular medicine, targeted therapies, and immunotherapy for a variety of cancers. Cutaneous lymphomas will be no exception. We all hope that over the next 10 years, we will build on our recent successes of the management of this complex disease.

Melbourne, VIC, Australia   H. Miles Prince, MD, FRACP, FRCPA

Preface

Despite being the most common form of cutaneous T-cell lymphoma, mycosis fungoides (MF) is a rare disease. Rare case presentation has limited research and the clinical knowledge of physicians. Furthermore, vague dermatologic symptoms have led to frequent misdiagnosis and ill management.

The goal of this book is to provide a comprehensive text that will enable the practicing physician to diagnose and stage MF as a cutaneous T-cell lymphoma upon presentation, and subsequently serve as a guide for proper treatment methods.

Written for dermatologists, oncologists, hematologists, internists, and family physicians, this book is divided into four parts: Overview of Disorder, Research Study, Case Reports, and Clinical Case Photos. Chapters in Part I include Introduction and History, Epidemiology, Etiology, Diagnosis and Management, Staging, Treatment, and Variants of Mycosis Fungoides. Each chapter is designed to provide insight and reference for clinicians with the addition of dozens of high-quality photographs from ten individual patients, illustrations, and clinical tables.

While the presentation of MF cases is uncommon, the disease's rarity has limited clinician knowledge of the disease. In order to adequately serve current patients and manage inevitable future patients with MF, *Clinician's Guide to Mycosis Fungoides* is the only book available that serves specifically as a comprehensive guide for physicians.

This book is a part of Clinician's Guide Series published by International Springer Publication. The Clinician's Guide Series focuses on various diseases with a high rate of misdiagnosis in order to provide the most comprehensive reference material for physicians, nurses, clinicians and students who are studying in medical and clinical fields. The intention of this series is to shed light on the research on the misdiagnosis of these diseases and the difficulties experienced in accurately diagnosing them.

A delay in accurate diagnosis and treatment has the potential to yield a less desirable case outcome for both the patients and the healthcare professionals who care for them. However, investing in this research is a milestone for fundamental changes in medicine and innovative decision making which could ameliorate or save the lives of countless patients.

Seattle, WA   Pooya Khan Mohammad Beigi

Acknowledgements

Special Thanks to:
Ashkan Emadi, MD
Anthony P. Cheung, MD
Joseph Connors, MD
Youwen Zhou, MD
Barry Kassen, MD
Jack Burak, MD
Michael Hamridge, MD
Mark Gaber, MD
Roy Colven, MD
Gary S. Wood, MD
Amirhosein Emami, MD
Shahin Akhondzadeh, MD
Nima Rezaie, MD
Hamed Hoseini, MD
Nafiseh Esmaeili, MD
Amirhoushang Ehsani, MD
Pedram Nourmohammadpour, MD
Minoo Mohraz, MD
Batool Rashidi, MD
Fatemeh Ghannadi, MD
Ahmad Jalili, MD
Franz Trautinger, MD
Deborah James

and

Misdiagnosis Association Research Assistants
Ashutosh Sharma
Dyviani Latchman
YiWeng Yang
Atefeh Sadiri
Arezoo Sadiri
Negin Askari
Tanya Dhami
Smruthi Ramachandran

Contents

Contributors

- **Pooya Khan Mohammad Beigi, MSc, MD, MPH** Department of Health Management, New York Medical College, Valhalla, NY, USA

  University of British Columbia, Vancouver, BC, Canada

  Misdiagnosis Association, Seattle, WA, USA
  The main author of all chapters

- **Hassan Seirafi, MD** Department of Dermatology, Tehran University of Medical Sciences, Tehran, Iran, Chapters: 8-24

- **Emanual Maverakis, MD** Department of Dermatology, University of California Davis, Sacramento, CA, USA, Chapters: 1-7

- **Seyed Sajad Niyyati, BS** Department of Biology, University of British Columbia, Vancouver, BC, Canada

  Misdiagnosis Association, Seattle, WA, USA, Chapters: 1-7

- **H. Miles Prince, MD, FRACP, FRCPA** Department of Hematology, University of Melbourne, Melbourne, VIC, Australia, Foreword

- **Elizabeth Alice Wang, BS, BA** Department of Dermatology, University of California Davis/UC Davis Medical Center, Sacramento, CA, USA, Chapters: 1-7

- **Mohammadreza Ataie, MD** Department of Dermatology, Tehran University of Medical Sciences, Tehran, Iran, Chapters: 8-13

- **Soneet Dhillon, BS** Department of Dermatology, University of California Davis, Sacramento, CA, USA, Chapters: 4-6

Part I

Overview of Disorder

Introduction and History

1

Mycosis fungoides (MF) is a mature non-Hodgkin lymphoma of T cell origin, and a type of cutaneous T cell lymphoma (CTCL). MF was first recognized in 1806 by a French dermatologist, Jean-Louis-Marc Alibert at the L'hôpital St. Louis in France [1]. In 1814, Alibert first named the disease pian fungoides due to its similarity with the treponemal disease yaws, or pian. In 1832, he went on to describe it as "a strange disorder of the skin with mushroom-like tumors" [2]. Alibert's patient at the time suffered from desquamating rashes, which progressed into multiple lesions on his face and trunk region. Although Alibert was not aware of MF's pathological background, he was aware that the lymphoma was indeed not a fungus [1].

In 1876, MF became known as Alibert-Bazin disease, named after Alibert and Pierre-Antoine-Ernest Bazin who contributed toward an early comprehensive characterization of the disease [1]. Their description of MF included three stages: nonspecific erythematous (premycotic), plaque (lichenoid), and tumor (fungoid). Bazin described a progression from premycotic phase to plaque lesions and finally to tumors. Following these discoveries, Vidal and Barocq described MF d'emblée for patients with tumors not preceded by plaques or patches (cases of which are now thought to represent other forms of CTCL). Besnier and Haopeau later characterized an erythrodermic form of MF [3, 4]. Taken together, these descriptions formed the early characterizations of MF, which were later followed by descriptions of Sézary's syndrome (SS), the leukemic variant of CTCL.

Today we know that CTCL comprise a diverse group of non-Hodgkin lymphomas (NHL) caused by malignant skin-trafficking T cells. MF is the most common type of CTCL. Primary cutaneous lymphomas are classified by the European Organization for Research and Treatment of Cancer (EORTC) and the World Health Organization (WHO) (Table 1.1).

MF is a mature T cell NHL that primarily develops in the skin, but can also involve lymph nodes, blood, and other organs. Clinically, MF typically begins as variably sized, pruritic, erythematous patches with a fine scale [5]. Although a small percentage of MF patients may progress to developing patches, nodules, and/or gradually enlarging tumors that can undergo necrosis and ulceration, most patients

© Springer International Publishing AG 2017
P.K.M. Beigi, *Clinician's Guide to Mycosis Fungoides*,
DOI 10.1007/978-3-319-47907-1_1

Table 1.1 Frequency of disease and 5-year survival rate obtained from the European Organization for Research and Treatment of Cancer (EORTC) and the World Health Organization (WHO)

Disease classification	Frequency (%)	5-Year survival rate (%)
Mycosis fungoides (MF)	54	88
Folliculotropic MF	6	80
Pagetoid reticulosis	1	100
Granulomatous slack skin	<1	100
Primary cutaneous anaplastic large cell lymphoma (C-ALCL)	10	95
Lymphomatoid papulosis (LyP)	16	100
Sézary syndrome (SS)	4	24
Extranodal NK/T-cell lymphoma, nasal type	1	<5

with MF do not progress beyond patch- or plaque-type disease [5]. Patients with MF typically have a prolonged clinical course.

Early lesions of MF may show variable degrees of epidermal atrophy, telangiectasia, and/or mottled hyper- or hypopigmentation. The term "poikoderma" refers to a combination of these features, the presence of which is highly suggestive of MF. These initial skin lesions have a tendency to asymmetrically affect the buttocks, trunks, and limbs. Patients often have nonspecific dermatitis and/or psoriasiform skin lesions for many years that are frequently misdiagnosed as atopic, contact, nummular, or photo-induced dermatitis (see Chap. 4 *Diagnosis and Differential Diagnosis* section). For these reasons and more, diagnosing early MF proves to be challenging.

Contributors to This Chapter

- Pooya Khan Mohammad Beigi, MD, University of British Columbia, BC, Canada
- Elizabeth Alice Wang, BS, University of California Davis, Sacramento, CA, USA
- Seyed Sajad Niyyati, BS, University of British Columbia, Vancouver, BC, Canada
- Emanual Maverakis, MD, University of California Davis, Sacramento, CA, USA

References

1. Karamanou M, Psaltopoulou T, Tsoucalas G, Androutsos G. Baron Jean-Louis Alibert (1768-1837) and the first description of mycosis fungoides. J BUON. 2014;19(2):585.
2. Wiernik PH. Neoplastic diseases of the blood. Cambridge: Cambridge University Press; 2003.

3. Vonderheid EC, Bernengo MG, Burg G, Duvic M, Heald P, Laroche L, et al. Update on erythrodermic cutaneous t-cell lymphoma: Report of the international society for cutaneous lymphomas. J Am Acad Dermatol. 2002;46(1):95–106.
4. Besnier E, Hallopeau H. On the erythrodermia of mycosis fungoides. J Cutan Genitourin Dis. 1892;10:453.
5. Ashton R, Leppard B. Differential diagnosis in dermatology. Oxford: Radcliffe; 2005.

Epidemiology

2

The overall age-adjusted incidence of mycosis fungoides (MF) worldwide is around 6–7 cases per 1 million [1]. MF is thought to be a disease of the elderly, as 75 % of cases are seen in the age group of 50–60 years [2]. However, MF can be seen in patients under the age of 35 years old with similar findings and clinical course [3]. MF has in fact been identified in children and teenagers [4]; 0.5–5 % of all cases are diagnosed before age 20 years [5, 6]. In addition, MF is observed more commonly in males than females, with a male-to-female ratio of 2:1 [5, 7]—a finding that is more pronounced in children. In a study looking at juvenile-onset MF, 24 out of 34 patients were male (74 %) [1].

In the United States, the incidence of MF, up until the year 2000, was reported to have increased over time [8], a phenomenon that may be reflective of improvements in diagnostics or reporting. Between 1973 and 2002, an increase in the incidence of MF was found to correlate with a higher density of medical specialists. However according to the Surveillance, Epidemiology, and End Results (SEER) registry data, the incidence of MF appears to have stabilized since then [9].

Contributors to This Chapter

- Pooya Khan Mohammad Beigi, MD, University of British Columbia, BC, Canada
- Elizabeth Alice Wang, BS, University of California Davis, Sacramento, CA, USA
- Seyed Sajad Niyyati, BS, University of British Columbia, Vancouver, BC, Canada
- Emanual Maverakis, MD, University of California Davis, Sacramento, CA, USA

© Springer International Publishing AG 2017
P.K.M. Beigi, *Clinician's Guide to Mycosis Fungoides*,
DOI 10.1007/978-3-319-47907-1_2

event in MF [14]. Since then, immunohistochemical studies have found that the neoplastic cells of MF—so-called mycosis cells (MCs) that are uniquely characterized by irregular, "cerebriform" nuclei—have been found to frequently co-occur with LCs in the epidermis of MF skin lesions, with LCs forming close epithelial-like contacts with MCs [15]. Phenotypic characterization of the cells has revealed that SS is a malignancy derived from the central memory T cells, while MF is of skin resident effector memory T cell origin [16]. Immunologically, neoplastic T cells in tumor stage MF has been shown to derive from CD4+ T cells with a Th2 cytokine profile, and an impaired Th1 cell-mediated antitumor response has also been implicated in MF [17, 18].

Contributors to This Chapter

- Pooya Khan Mohammad Beigi, MD, University of British Columbia, BC, Canada
- Elizabeth Alice Wang, BS, University of California Davis, Sacramento, CA, USA
- Seyed Sajad Niyyati, BS, University of British Columbia, Vancouver, BC, Canada
- Emanual Maverakis, MD, University of California Davis, Sacramento, CA, USA

References

1. Sommer V, Clemmensen O, Nielsen O, Wasik M, Lovato P, Brender C, et al. In vivo activation of stat3 in cutaneous t-cell lymphoma. Evidence for an antiapoptotic function of stat3. Leukemia. 2004;18(7):1288–95.
2. Scarisbrick JJ, Woolford AJ, Russell-Jones R, Whittaker SJ. Loss of heterozygosity on 10q and microsatellite instability in advanced stages of primary cutaneous T-cell lymphoma and possible association with homozygous deletion of PTEN. Blood. 2000;95(9):2937–42.
3. Navas IC, Ortiz-Romero PL, Villuendas R, Martínez P, García C, Gómez E, et al. P16 ink4a gene alterations are frequent in lesions of mycosis fungoides. Am J Pathol. 2000;156(5):1565–72.
4. Tracey L, Villuendas R, Dotor AM, Spiteri I, Ortiz P, García JF, et al. Mycosis fungoides shows concurrent deregulation of multiple genes involved in the TNF signaling pathway: an expression profile study. Blood. 2003;102(3):1042–50.
5. Tan RH, Butterworth C, McLaughlin H, Malka S, Samman P. Mycosis fungoides—a disease of antigen persistence. Br J Dermatol. 1974;91(6):607–16.
6. Girardi M, Heald PW, Wilson LD. The pathogenesis of mycosis fungoides. N Engl J Med. 2004;350(19):1978–88.
7. Gemmill R, editor. Cutaneous T-cell lymphoma. Seminars in oncology nursing. Amsterdam: Elsevier; 2006.
8. Whittemore AS, Holly EA, Lee I-M, Abel EA, Adams RM, Nickoloff BJ, et al. Mycosis fungoides in relation to environmental exposures and immune response: a case-control study. J Natl Cancer Inst. 1989;81(20):1560–7.
9. Ghosh SK, Abrams J, Terunuma H, Vonderheid EC, DeFreitas E. Human T-cell leukemia virus type I tax/rex DNA and RNA in cutaneous T-cell lymphoma. Blood. 1994;84(8):2663–71.

10. Wood GS, Salvekar A, Schaffer J, Crooks CF, Henghold W, Fivenson DP, et al. Evidence against a role for human T-cell lymphotrophic virus type I (HTLV-I) in the pathogenesis of American cutaneous T-cell lymphoma. J Invest Dermatol. 1996;107(3):301–7.

11. Wood GS, Schaffer JM, Boni R, Dummer R, Burg G, Takeshita M, et al. No evidence of HTLV-I proviral integration in lymphoproliferative disorders associated with cutaneous T-cell lymphoma. Am J Pathol. 1997;150(2):667.

12. Pancake BA, Zucker-Franklin D, Coutavas EE. The cutaneous T cell lymphoma, mycosis fungoides, is a human T cell lymphotropic virus-associated disease. A study of 50 patients. J Clin Investig. 1995;95(2):547.

13. Zucker-Franklin D, Pancake BA, editors. The role of human T-cell lymphotropic viruses (HTLV-I and II) in cutaneous T-cell lymphomas. Seminars in dermatology; 1994.

14. Rowden G, Lewis M. Langerhans cells: involvement in the pathogenesis of mycosis fungoides. Br J Dermatol. 1976;95(6):665–72.

15. Bani D, Pimpinelli N, Moretti S, Giannotti B. Langerhans cells and mycosis fungoides–a critical overview of their pathogenic role in the disease. Clin Exp Dermatol. 1990;15(1):7–12.

16. Campbell JJ, Clark RA, Watanabe R, Kupper TS. Sezary syndrome and mycosis fungoides arise from distinct T-cell subsets: a biologic rationale for their distinct clinical behaviors. Blood. 2010;116(5):767–71.

17. Kim EJ, Hess S, Richardson SK, Newton S, Showe LC, Benoit BM, et al. Immunopathogenesis and therapy of cutaneous T cell lymphoma. J Clin Invest. 2005;115(4):798–812.

18. Vowels BR, Cassin M, Vonderheid EC, Rook AH. Aberrant cytokine production by Sezary syndrome patients: cytokine secretion pattern resembles murine th2 cells. J Invest Dermatol. 1992;99(1):90–4.

Diagnosis and Management

4

Clinical Features

Although the "Alibert–Bazin" (often referred to as "classical" in many texts) type of mycosis fungoides (MF) is typically characterized by progressive stages of patches, plaques, and tumors, as was initially described in 1876, patients with MF commonly demonstrate a chronic, indolent clinical course over years, possibly decades, and many patients in fact do not demonstrate a progression beyond the plaque stage. A "premycotic" period often precedes a definite diagnosis of MF, during which patients may have nonspecific, chronic, finely scaling lesions that may wax and wane over years, which may result in nondiagnostic biopsies. These lesions can also clinically resemble common skin conditions such as eczema, psoriasis, or drug reactions and thus may be misdiagnosed early in the course of the disease (see next section: "Diagnosis and Differential Diagnosis"). For these reasons, patients with early stages of MF presenting with these nonspecific dermatoses can have lesions for some length of time before a definitive diagnosis can be made.

Early MF lesions commonly present as scaly patches that are variable in size, shape, color, pigmentation (hyper- and hypo-), and degree of epidermal atrophy. These lesions can be pruritic and preferentially affect the buttocks and truncal areas [1]. Women frequently display the first signs of MF in their buttocks, thighs, and breasts. Patches may evolve into plaques, which have a more generalized distribution, and annular or arciform configuration. Plaque lesions also have a more infiltrated reddish-brown appearance.

A small percentage of patients will progress to developing firm, violaceous nodules and/or exophytic tumors, which can undergo necrosis and ulceration. Lymphadenopathy may be appreciated on physical exam in this stage. Extensive tumors and indurated plaques affecting the face may result in prominent brows and leonine facies. These lesions can also be found in uncommon sites such as the oral and genital mucosae [2]. In the late stage disease, confluence of lesions may result in erythroderma.

P.K.M. Beigi, *Clinician's Guide to Mycosis Fungoides*,
DOI 10.1007/978-3-319-47907-1_4

Generalized erythroderma represents more advanced disease, in which patients can have generalized, severe skin involvement with intense pruritus and scaling. Cutaneous manifestations in the tumor and erythroderma stages of MF can be intensely symptomatic. Luckily, the majority of patients do not progress to have this advanced cutaneous disease. Of note, erythroderma is also a characteristic feature of the aggressive leukemic cutaneous T cell lymphoma (CTCL) variant, Sézary syndrome (SS). In rare cases, SS may follow classic MF. However, SS is considered separate from MF [3]. Erythrodermic MF is distinguished from SS insofar as the former has absent/minimal blood involvement, whereas SS is characterized by circulating atypical T cells (Sézary cells).

Diagnosis and Differential Diagnosis

MF has been said to mimic more than 50 different clinical entities [4]. The differential for the scaling patches and plaques seen in MF is broad. The lesions in MF commonly resemble other skin disorders such as eczema, psoriasis, parapsoriasis, superficial fungal infections, photodermatitis, and drug reactions—although a thorough examination of histologic features and skin findings can generally exclude these diagnoses. A solitary MF lesion can resemble nummular eczema, lichen simplex chronicus, erythema chronicum migrans, and tinea corporis [5]. In addition, tumorous lesions in MF can mimic those of other cutaneous lymphomas. Erythrodermic MF can resemble generalized atopic dermatitis, erythrodermic psoriasis, and contact dermatitis.

For these reasons and more, diagnostic algorithms have been generated to facilitate an accurate diagnosis of MF. The International Society for Cutaneous Lymphomas (ISCL) has proposed a point-based algorithm for the diagnosis of early MF, which incorporates clinical, histopathologic, molecular biologic, and immunopathologic criteria as outlined in Table 4.1 [5].

Workup for Suspected Mycosis Fungoides

A full history and physical, with attention to skin and percent body surface area (BSA), peripheral lymph nodes, and organomegaly/masses (spleen/liver) should be performed in the clinical evaluation for suspected MF.

Important studies to perform in the workup of MF include biopsies of the skin and suspicious lymph nodes, if applicable, in order to yield a pathologic diagnosis. Laboratory studies and imaging may be necessary to allow for an evaluation of tumor burden and staging. The need for further examinations and studies, as well as treatment options, is dependent on the stage of the disease (see Chaps. 5 and 6 on Staging and Treatment).

Table 4.1 A point-based algorithm for the diagnosis of early MF, incorporating clinical, histopathologic, molecular biologic, and immunopathologic criteria (Adapted from the International Society for Cutaneous Lymphomas [5])

Criteria	Major (2 points)	Minor (1 point)
Clinical		
Persistent and/or progressive patches and plaques plus:	Any 2	Any 1
1. Non-sun-exposed location		
2. Size/shape variation		
3. Poikiloderma		
Histopathologic		
Superficial lymphoid infiltrate plus:	Both	Either
1. Epidermotropism without spongiosis		
2. Lymphoid atypia		
Molecular/biologic: clonal TCR gene rearrangement	NA	Present
Immunopathologic		
1. CD2,3,5 less than 50% of T cells	NA	Present
2. CD7 less than 10% of T cells		
3. Epidermal discordance from expression of CD2, 3, 5 of CD7 on dermal T cells		

Pathology

Biopsy of suspicious skin sites followed by dermatopathologic review is essential in the diagnosis of MF, which can be followed up with immunophenotyping, genetic testing, and/or molecular analysis of skin biopsy in search of clonal T-cell rearrangements [6]. As indicated in the point-based diagnostic algorithm outlined in Table 4.1, a diagnosis of MF is more likely if flow cytometry demonstrates an aberrant immunophenotype, i.e., loss of one or more T-cell-associated antigens such as CD7. A diagnosis of MF is also more likely if clonal TCR gene rearrangement is present, although these should be interpreted with caution since these can be found in nonmalignant conditions or may not be demonstrated in all cases of MF [6].

The diagnosis of early MF is challenging due to its similarity with other inflammatory diseases even at the histological level. Microscopic findings of early MF can be nonspecific and overlap with other inflammatory or benign diseases, which can result in nondiagnostic biopsies. Nonetheless, important differentiating features have been identified. In 1979 Sanchez and Ackerman highlighted changes occurring in the epidermis of MF that could be distinguished from those occurring in spongiotic inflammatory disorders [7], and found an increased number of intraepidermal lymphocytes in MF (epidermatotropism) [8]. They also reported that an increase in intercellular spaces between keratinocytes is also seen in MF, but argued that spongiotic microvesiculation is not, the presence of which would indicate a spongiotic dermatosis [8]. Another important observation was that these intraepidermal cells appeared to be surrounded by vacuolated halos. Sanchez and Ackerman also posited that while these atypical lymphocytes may not be found in the earliest lesions of MF, they can be found in later stages of the disease [8].

Since then, observations following this seminal discovery have corroborated these findings and expanded our current understanding of the histological features of early patch MF. In 1988, Nickoloff demonstrated that the basal layers of the epidermis in MF are linearly lined with lymphocytes [9]. We now know that patch MF is indeed characterized by atypical lymphocytes that form band-like or lichenoid infiltrates along the edges of the basal layer. A later finding by King-Ismael and Ackerman described lymphocytes within the epidermis that were larger than those present in the dermis [10]. They also reported the presence of papillary dermal fibrosis associated with a patchy lichenoid lymphocytic infiltrate. Biopsies have shown that a key differentiating factor of early MF is the presence of medium to large lymphocytes with convoluted nuclei within the epidermis, which are larger lymphocytes than those seen in inflammatory dermatoses. These atypical cells are mycosis cells, which are mature skin-homing CD4+ T cells. Epidermotropism of this infiltrate of T lymphocytes is a key finding, and they can form microabscesses in the epidermis, Pautrier's microabscesses [2].

When this T-cell infiltrate in the epidermis proliferates, which extends deep into the dermis and beyond, the patchy lesions of MF advance to the plaque and tumor stages. In the plaque stage of MF, the epidermis is thickened and can exhibit a psoriasiform pattern but with rare or absent spongiosis. In the plaque stage of MF, it is not uncommon to find dermal infiltrates comprised of atypical cells with irregular cerebriform nuclei [2]. In the tumor stage of MF, both the upper dermis and lower dermis contain dense dermal infiltrates of medium- and large-sized cerebriform lymphocytes. Importantly, at this stage there may be a loss of epidermotropism.

It is to be noted that the immunohistochemical features of the leukemic variant of MF, Sézary syndrome (SS), may be similar to those of MF with the following key differences: (1) more monotonous cellular infiltrates in SS; (2) possibly absent epidermotropism; and (3) increased lymph node involvement with dense infiltrates of Sézary cells, which are characteristic pleomorphic malignant T cells. Sézary cells also characteristically have cerebriform nuclei, and traffic to the skin, lymph nodes, and peripheral blood. Diagnosis of SS requires demonstration of a T-cell clone in the peripheral blood, and of an expanded CD4 T cell population, and Sézary cell count of at least 1000 cells per μ(mu)L [11].

Laboratory Studies

The following laboratory tests are included in the diagnosis of MF [6, 12]:

1. Comprehensive metabolic panel (CMP) and complete blood count (CBC) with differential. A manual slide review should be undertaken for Sézary cells ("Sézary cell prep"). The detection of Sézary cells in the peripheral blood is primarily based on morphological features such as cerebriform nuclei.

2. Liver function tests are necessary to assess for extracutaneous manifestations of MF, which are uncommon but can include involvement of the liver.
3. Uric acid and lactate dehydrogenase level can serve as markers of bulky and/or biologically aggressive disease.
4. Flow cytometric study of the blood (include available T cell-related antibodies) is needed to detect a circulating malignant clone.
5. TCR gene rearrangement of peripheral blood lymphocytes if blood involvement is suspected.
6. Consider human immunodeficiency virus (HIV) and human T-lymphotropic virus types 1 (HTLV-1) testing, especially if the patient is from an endemic region (Japan, Caribbean). HTLV-1 has been reported in the peripheral blood and/or cutaneous lesions of some patients with MF.

Imaging Studies

For early MF, posteroanterior (PA) and lateral chest radiographs is warranted, and peripheral nodal chains can be assessed with ultrasound. For stages greater than IIA, a chest/abdominal/pelvic contrast-enhanced computed tomography (CT) scan should be undertaken and positron emission tomography (PET)-CT can be considered [6, 13].

Contributors to This Chapter

- Pooya Khan Mohammad Beigi, MD, University of British Columbia, BC, Canada
- Elizabeth Alice Wang, BS, University of California Davis, Sacramento, CA, USA
- Seyed Sajad Niyyati, BS, University of British Columbia, Vancouver, BC, Canada
- Soneet Dhillon, BS, University of California Davis, Sacramento, CA, USA
- Emanual Maverakis, MD, University of California Davis, Sacramento, CA, USA

References

1. Jawed SI, Myskowski PL, Horwitz S, Moskowitz A, Querfeld C. Primary cutaneous T-cell lymphoma (mycosis fungoides and sezary syndrome): Part II. Prognosis, management, and future directions. J Am Acad Dermatol. 2014;70(2):223e221–3, e217.
2. Yamashita T, Abbade LPF, Marques MEA, Marques SA. Mycosis fungoides and sézary syndrome: clinical, histopathological and immunohistochemical review and update. An Bras Dermatol. 2012;87(6):817–30.
3. Cerroni L, Gatter K, Kerl H. Front matter. Wiley Online Library; 2009.
4. Nashan D, Faulhaber D, Ständer S, Luger T, Stadler R. Mycosis fungoides: a dermatological masquerader. Br J Dermatol. 2007;156(1):1–10.

5. Pimpinelli N, Olsen EA, Santucci M, Vonderheid E, Haeffner AC, Stevens S, et al. Defining early mycosis fungoides. J Am Acad Dermatol. 2005;53(6):1053–63.
6. National Comprehensive Cancer Network. NCCN clinical practice guidelines in oncology: non-Hodgkin's lymphoma version 3 (2016), Vol. 3. Fort Washington: National Comprehensive Care Network; 2016. p. 105–18.
7. Sanchez JL, Ackerman BA. The patch stage of mycosis fungoides criteria for histologic diagnosis. Am J Dermatopathol. 1979;1(1):5.
8. Harvey NT, Spagnolo DV, Wood BA. 'Could it be mycosis fungoides?': An approach to diagnosing patch stage mycosis fungoides. J Hematopathol. 2015;8(4):209–23.
9. Nickoloff BJ. Light-microscopic assessment of 100 patients with patch/plaque-stage mycosis fungoides. Am J Dermatopathol. 1988;10(5):469–77.
10. King-Ismael D, Ackerman AB. Guttate parapsoriasis/digitate dermatosis (small plaque parapsoriasis) is mycosis fungoides. Am J Dermatopathol. 1992;14(6):518–30.
11. Vonderheid EC, Kotecha A, Boselli CM, Bigler RD, Lessin SR, Bernengo MG, et al. Variable CD7 expression on T cells in the leukemic phase of cutaneous T cell lymphoma (sezary syndrome). J Invest Dermatol. 2001;117(3):654–62.
12. Mori M. New xenon-chloride lamp useful for treating early-stage mycosis fungoides. J Am Acad Dermatol. 2004;50:943–5.
13. Galper SL, Smith BD, Wilson LD. Diagnosis and management of mycosis fungoides. Oncology. 2010;24(6):491.

Staging

5

Staging of mycosis fungoides (MF) can be done through the TNMB (tumor-node-metastasis-blood) classification system put forth by the National Comprehensive Cancer Network (NCCN) and is best summarized in Table 5.1. The TNMB system stages the disease based on the extent of skin, lymph node, viscera, and blood involvement. Of note, stages IA to IIA are also referred to as early MF. Advanced stage is IIB to IV.

In the TNMB system, T represents the extent of skin involvement, ranging from T1 to T4 based on severity. Lymph node involvement is represented by N and ranges from N0 to N3, with NX representing abnormal nodes without histological confirmation. Visceral organ involvement is classified into M in which M0 represents no visceral involvement, and M1 represents confirmed visceral involvement. MX represents abnormal viscera with no histological confirmation. Blood involvement is classified into B; the degree of blood involvement ranges from B0 in which there is no blood involvement, to B2 in which there is a high blood tumor burden. The TNMB stages can then be translated into clinical stages IA through IVB (Table 5.2) [1].

Stage IA is generally defined as presence of limited patches, plaques, and or papules covering less than 10 % of the skin surface (T1) and may include low to no blood tumor burden (B0, B1). Once the patches, plaques, and or papules cover more than 10 % of the skin surface (T2), the cancer is staged as IB.

The presence of abnormal lymph nodes scoring histopathology Dutch Gr 1–2 (N1, N2) is indicative of stage IIA. Once 1 or more tumors greater than 1 cm in diameter are present (T3), the patient is then stage IIB. The cancer is staged as IIIA when there is a confluence of erythema covering greater than 80 % of the body surface area (T4). If there is a low blood tumor burden (B1), the cancer is staged as IIIB.

A high blood tumor burden (B2) indicates stage IV disease, even if lymph nodes score histopathology Dutch Gr 2 or below (N0–N2). Abnormal lymph nodes scoring histopathology Dutch Gr 3 without the involvement of viscera (M0) are classified as IVA$_2$. The involvement of viscera (M1) stages the cancer as IVB [2].

© Springer International Publishing AG 2017

P.K.M. Beigi, *Clinician's Guide to Mycosis Fungoides*,
DOI 10.1007/978-3-319-47907-1_5

Table 5.1 Classification staging of mycosis fungoides

TNMB	Classification Staging of Mycosis Fungoides and Sézary Syndrome
T1	Limited patches, papules, and/or plaques covering < 10% of the skin
T2	Papules, patches, and/or plaques covering ≥ 10% of the skin
T3	One or more tumors (≥ 1 cm in diameter)
T4	Confluence of erythema ≥ 80% of body surface area
N0	No biopsy required, no abnormal lymph nodes
N1	Abnormal lymph nodes; histopathology Dutch Gr 1 or NCI LN 0-2
N2	Abnormal lymph nodes; histopathology Dutch Gr 2 or NCI LN 3
N3	Abnormal lymph nodes; histopathology Dutch Gr 3-4 or NCI LN 4
NX	Abnormal lymph nodes; histopathology Dutch Gr 1 or NCI LN 0-2
M0	No visceral organ involvement
M1	Visceral organ involvement with pathology confirmation
MX	Abnormal visceral site without histological confirmation
B0	Absence of significant blood involvement with ≤ 5% peripheral blood lymphocytes are Sézary cells
B1	Low blood tumor burden: > 5% of peripheral blood lymphocytes are Sézary cells. Does not meet criteria of B2
B2	≥ 1000/mcL Sézary cells or CD4/CD8 ≥ 10 or ≥ 40% CD4+/CD7- or ≥ 30% CD4+/CD26- cells

TNMB - tumor-node-metastasis-blood

Adapted from the National Comprehensive Cancer Network Guidelines for non-Hodgkin lymphomas
TNMB tumor-node-metastasis-blood

Contributors to This Chapter

- Pooya Khan Mohammad Beigi, MD, University of British Columbia, BC, Canada
- Elizabeth Alice Wang, BS, University of California Davis, Sacramento, CA, USA
- Seyed Sajad Niyyati, BS, University of British Columbia, Vancouver, BC, Canada
- Soneet Dhillon, BS, University of California Davis, Sacramento, CA, USA
- Emanual Maverakis, MD, University of California Davis, Sacramento, CA, USA

Table 5.2 Clinical staging
of mycosis fungoides and
Sézary syndrome

	Tumor	Node	Metastasis	Blood
IA	1	0	0	0,1
IB	2	0	0	0,1
IIA	1-2	1,2	0	0,1
IIB	3	0-2	0	0,1
IIIA	4	0-2	0	0
IIIB	4	0-2	0	1
IVA$_1$	1-4	0-2	0	2
IVA$_2$	1-4	3	0	0-2
IVB	1-4	0-3	1	0-2

Adapted from the National Comprehensive
Cancer Network Guidelines for NHL

References

1. National Comprehensive Cancer Network. NCCN clinical practice guidelines in oncology: non-Hodgkin's lymphoma version 3 (2016), Vol. 3. Fort Washington: National Comprehensive Care Network; 2016. p. 105–18.
2. Ashton R, Leppard B. Differential diagnosis in dermatology. Oxford: Radcliffe; 2005.

Treatment

6

Treatment of mycosis fungoides (MF) depends in large part on the stage of the disease. Consensus recommendations on the treatment of MF have been proposed by several organizations, and those put forth by the National Comprehensive Cancer Network (NCCN) form the basis of this chapter. These recommendations are stage-based algorithms. They include management recommendations based on response to therapy at particular stages of the disease (Stage IA–Stage IV), i.e., whether or not the patient has a complete response (CR), a partial response (PR), inadequate response, refractory disease, or progression of the disease. A CR is one that results in complete disappearance of all clinical evidence of disease, while PR is one that results in regression of disease [1].

The NCCN treatment guidelines and algorithms also provide recommendations for disease management in the case of histologic evidence of folliculotropic or large-cell transformed MF. Management differs in these cases, as typical MF can occasionally transform into a large cell lymphoma, a diagnosis that carries a worse prognosis (median survival as low as 1–2 years). Folliculotropic MF is a variant of MF (described in Chap. 7: Variants of MF) and is a distinct disease entity that also has different management guidelines.

In general, treatment options for MF include skin-directed therapies, systemic therapies, and combination therapies. Skin-directed therapies include topical corticosteroids, topical chemotherapy, local radiation, topical retinoids, total skin electron beam therapy (TSEBT), phototherapy (ultraviolet B, psoralen, and ultraviolet A), and topical imiquimod. Systemic therapies are summarized in Table 6.1. Systemic therapies are used in advanced or refractory stages of MF [2]. Combination therapies are those that combine skin-directed therapies and systemic therapies, or various types of systemic therapies.

Patients with skin-limited disease may only require topical therapy to induce remission. Ultimately, the method of treatment used for MF depends not only on the stage of the disease, but also the availability of the treatment, and patient and physician preference (Figs. 6.1, 6.2, 6.3, 6.4, and 6.5).

© Springer International Publishing AG 2017
P.K.M. Beigi, *Clinician's Guide to Mycosis Fungoides*,
DOI 10.1007/978-3-319-47907-1_6

Table 6.1 Overview of treatment regimens

Skin-Directed Therapies	Systemic Therapies	Combination Therapies

LIMITED/LOCALIZED SKIN INVOLVEMENT
• Topical corticosteroids
• Topical chemotherapy
   › Mechlorethamine
   › Nitrogen mustard
   › Carmustine
• Local radiation
• Topical retinoids
• Phototherapy
   › UVB
   › nbUVB for patch/thin plaques
   › PUVA for thicker plaques
• Topical imiquimod
 	
GENERALIZED SKIN INVOLVEMENT
• Topical corticosteroids
• Topical chemotherapy
   › Mechlorethamine
   › Nitrogen mustard
   › Carmustine
• Phototherapy
   › UVB
   › nbUVB for patch/thin plaques
   › PUVA for thicker plaques
• Total skin electron beam therapy (TSEBT) for those with severe skin symptoms or generalized thick plaque or tumors, or poor response to other therapies
	CATEGORY A
	• Retinoids
	   › Bexarotene
	   › All-trans retinoic acid
	   › Isotretinoin
	    (13-cis-retinoic acid)
	• Interferons
	   › IFN-alpha
	   › IFN-gamma
	• HDAC-inhibitors
	   › Vorinostat
	   › Romidepsin
	• Extracorporeal photopheresis
	   › UVB
	   › nbUVB for patch/thin plaques
	   › PUVA for thicker plaques
	• Methotrexate (≤100mg q week)
	
	CATEGORY B
	• First-line therapies
	   › Liposomal doxorubicin
	   › Gemcitabine
	• Second-line therapies
	   › Chlorambucil
	   › Pentostatin
	   › Etoposide
	   › Cyclophosphamide
	   › Temozolomide
	   › Methotrexate(>100mg q week)
	   › Low-dose pralatrexate
	
	CATEGORY C
	• Liposomal doxorubicin
	• Gemcitabin
	• Romidepsin
	• Low-or standard-dose pralatrexate
		SKIN-DIRECTED + SYSTEMIC
		• Phototherapy + retinoid
		• Photothreapy + IFN
		• Phototherpy + photopheresis
		• Total skin electron beam + photopheresis
		
		SYSTEMIC + SYSTEMIC
		• Retinoid + IFN
		• Photopheresis + retinoid
		• Photopheresis + IFN
		• Photopheresis + retinoid + IFN

Adapted from the National Comprehensive Cancer Network Guidelines for non-Hodgkin lymphomas
UVB ultraviolet B, *NB-UVB* narrow band ultraviolet B, *PUVA* psoralen plus ultraviolet A, *IFN* interferon, *HDAC* histone deacetylase

Skin-Directed Therapies

Skin-directed therapy is the cornerstone of MF management and includes the following broad modalities: topical agents, phototherapy, and local radiation with X-ray or total skin electron beam therapy (TSEBT).

Topical agents can be further broken down into the following specific therapies:

Topical Corticosteroids

Topical corticosteroids are effective in controlling disease activity of early MF, which is characterized by papules, patches, or plaques with limited, if any, lymph node involvement and no visceral involvement. In a study done by Zackheim et al.

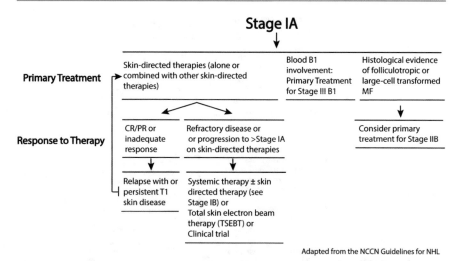

Fig. 6.1 Stage IA treatment algorithm. *CR* complete response, *PR* partial response, *MF* mycosis fungoides. Adapted from the National Comprehensive Cancer Network Guidelines for non-Hodgkin lymphomas

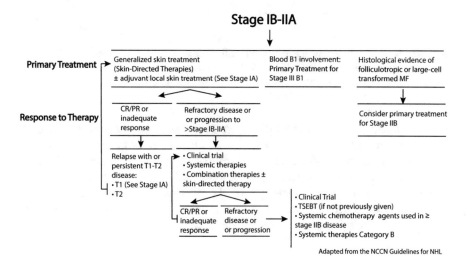

Fig. 6.2 Stage IB–IIA treatment algorithm. *CR* complete response, *PR* partial response, *MF* mycosis fungoides, *TSEBT* total skin electron beam. Adapted from the National Comprehensive Cancer Network Guidelines for non-Hodgkin lymphomas

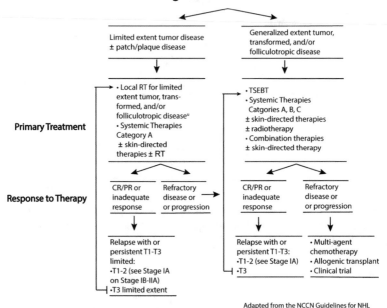

Fig. 6.3 Stage IIB treatment algorithm. *RT* radiotherapy, *CR* complete response, *PR* partial response, *MF* mycosis fungoides, *TSEBT* total skin electron beam. Adapted from the National Comprehensive Cancer Network Guidelines for non-Hodgkin lymphomas

with 79 patients, 63 % of patients with stage T1 disease who were treated with topical steroids demonstrated complete remission, while 31 % showed partial remission [2]. This study alone showed a 94 % total response rate in patients treated with topical steroids. However, persistent application can lead to skin atrophy and telangiectasias [3]. In more advanced stages of the disease or treatment-resistant MF, including tumor-stage plaques and nodules, topical steroids are used as adjuvant therapy, and intralesional corticosteroids can be used for thicker MF lesions [4].

Topical Chemotherapy

Chemotherapeutic agents used in MF include mechlorethamine (nitrogen mustard or HN_2) and carmustine (BCNU), both of which have proven to be safe and effective in controlling disease activity, particularly in early MF.

Nitrogen mustard is an alkylating agent and can be used as an initial therapy for treatment of MF patches and plaques. In a study of 76 patients studied over a 4-year period who were treated with HN_2, 50 % were free of detectable disease [5].

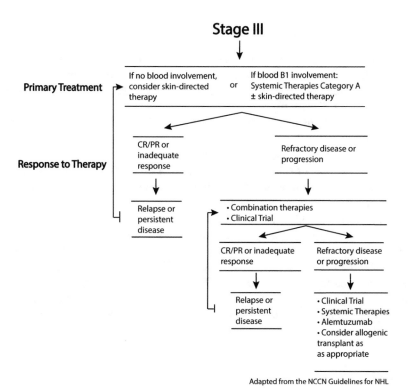

Fig. 6.4 Stage III treatment algorithm. *CR* complete response, *PR* partial response. Adapted from the National Comprehensive Cancer Network Guidelines for non-Hodgkin lymphomas

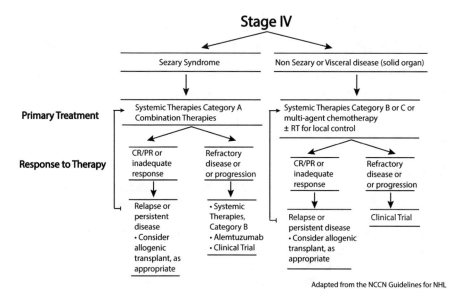

Fig. 6.5 Stage IV treatment algorithm. *RT* radiotherapy, *CR* complete response, *PR* partial response. Adapted from the National Comprehensive Cancer Network Guidelines for non-Hodgkin lymphomas

It is available as either ointment or aqueous formulation. Studies on MF patients treated with nitrogen mustard have demonstrated a 65 % complete response rate, 45 % 10-year relapse-free survival, and 95 % 10-year disease-specific survival in patients with T1 disease [6].

Side effects of this therapy include skin irritation, xerosis, hyperpigmentation, and, in rare cases, bullous reactions, urticarial rashes, and Stevens–Johnson syndrome [3, 7]. Long-term use has also been reported to be associated with increased risk for development of skin cancer. However, in a study of 203 patients with stages I–III MF treated with topical nitrogen mustard as monotherapy, the incidence of nonmelanoma skin cancers in patients who use topical nitrogen mustard is extremely low and occurred in only 2 (1 %) patients [6].

Topical carmustine (BCNU) has also been shown to be effective for early stage MF, with complete response rates of 92 % in stage T1 disease (less than 10 % skin involvement) and 64 % in stage T2 disease [8]. The 5-year relapse-free survival rate was reported to be 35 % and 10 % for T1 and T2 patients, respectively [9]. Side effects of this treatment include erythema, telangiectasias, and irritant or allergic dermatitis [10]. It is important to monitor complete blood count (CBC) as treatment with BCNU can also result in myelosuppression [11].

Topical Retinoids

Bexarotene has been approved by the US Food and Drug Administration (FDA) as a treatment option for early MF, in particular in those with refractory or persistent disease [2, 3]. Mechanistically, bexarotene is a rexinoid, a vitamin A-derived compound that binds to retinoid X receptors and ultimately alters gene transcription to enhance tumor apoptosis [12]. In patients with stage IA–IIA disease, application of topical bexarotene resulted in a response rate of 63 % and a complete clinical response of 21 % [13]. Complete clearance may take up to 16 weeks [14]. This therapy is generally well tolerated. Common side effects include pruritus, erythema, photosensitivity, and burning pain at the application site.

Light Therapy

Ultraviolet light, including ultraviolet B (UVB), narrow band UVB (NB-UVB), and psoralen plus ultraviolet A (PUVA) are also used in the treatment of MF. PUVA first appeared in 1976 and is one of the skin-directed therapies commonly used in the treatment of stages IA, IB, and IIA MF [15]. PUVA can result in total skin clearance and long-term remission [15], with complete response rates of up to 90 %, and has become a standard therapy for the early stages of MF [16].

UVB can be broadband, ranging from 290 to 320 nm, or narrowband ranging from 311 to 312 nm. UVB is generally used to treat thin patches and plaques, as UVB rays have limited penetration [3]. PUVA (psoralen plus UVA) differs from UVB in a variety of ways. First, UVA penetrates deeper into the skin in comparison to UVB, and thus has improved efficacy for thicker plaques. Also, in PUVA, prior to receiving UVA phototherapy, patients receive a skin-sensitizing medication by mouth, 8-methoxypsoralen. Intercalation of psoralen into DNA preempts the cells to undergo apoptosis upon exposure to UVA, which crosslinks the psoralen with the DNA. Of note, 8-methoxypsoralen is associated with side effects such as nausea and vomiting, and with enough treatments, skin cancer [3, 11]. Both UVB and PUVA are given to the patients 2–3 times per week, and the dose is increased based upon the patients' skin type until a complete response is achieved [11]. Once complete response is reached, PUVA can be given once every 2–4 weeks for several years on a maintenance basis [3].

Side effects associated with PUVA and UVB include skin erythema, hyperpigmentation, xerosis, pruritus, and even blistering. Long-term risks of phototherapy include photoaging and increased risk of melanoma and nonmelanoma skin cancers [11]. As such, phototherapy may not be appropriate in those with a history of UV-associated skin cancers.

PUVA can be used as a monotherapy or combination therapy. PUVA has been shown to result in higher response rates when combined with interferon alpha (IFN-α[alpha]). In early stage MF, PUVA in combination with IFN-α(alpha) has been associated with 100 % complete response rate [17]. Combination therapy has important implications for the tumor stage of MF, a stage that has been shown to be less responsive to PUVA monotherapy [2]. Another advantage of combination therapy is that the dosage of PUVA can be reduced to mitigate side effects. PUVA can also be combined with retinoids (RePUVA).

Total Skin Electron Beam Therapy

Radiotherapy (RT) can treat MF in the form of total skin electron beam therapy (TSEBT) and has been shown to be an effective treatment modality for stages T1–4 of MF [2]. In general, however, TSEBT is reserved for treatment-resistant disease, or those with severe skin symptoms or generalized thick plaque or tumors [18]. In a typical session, the patient receives 4–6 MeV of energy. A total dose of radiation over 30 Gy is typically necessary to achieve complete response [2]. The patient then receives fractions of dose of 1.5–2 Gy for about 8–10 weeks. It is also common practice to follow treatment with TSEBT with a systemic therapy as maintenance therapy [18].

For limited patches and plaques, TSEBT produces complete response rates of approximately 90 % [19]. In patients with tumor-stage disease, complete response rates of up to 40 % have been reported [3]. Side effects of TSEBT include alopecia, erythema, desquamation, xerosis, onychomadesis, and anhidrosis, which can persist for 6–12 months following treatment [2].

Radiotherapy can also be locally administered through X-ray or electron beam and can be used for those with single tumors or in combination with other modalities such as PUVA or photopheresis [18]. Photopheresis is a type of pheresis, also termed extracorporeal photochemotherapy (ECP), in which a patient's blood is

removed in aliquots, treated with a photosensitizing agent, and subjected to ultraviolet A light. This modality is classified as a type of systemic therapy and may
be more appropriate in patients with some blood involvement, i.e., B1 or B2 disease [18].

Topical Imiquimod

Topical imiquimod 5 % cream has been shown to result in a clinical response
rate of 50 % [20]. Imiquimod is a topically active immunomodulator that can
stimulate the production of IFN-alpha and various other cytokines. Case reports
have demonstrated it to be effective in the clearance of treatment-resistant
plaques [21].

Systemic Therapies

Systemic Retinoids

Systemic (oral) retinoids result in response rates of about 50 % in MF [22].
Isotretinoin (13-cis retinoic acid) and acitretin are examples of retinoids [11]. These
drugs and their metabolites act as agonists of the retinoic acid receptor (RAR) and
retinoid X receptor (RXR) nuclear receptors. The drugs are known to interrupt cell
differentiation and proliferation of cancerous cells, induce apoptosis, and fragment
DNA of sensitive T cell lines [23]. Retinoids can also be used in combination with
IFN-α(alpha) and PUVA [11]. The most common adverse effects of retinoids
include headaches, diminished night vision, photosensitivity, xerosis, elevated
transaminases, and hyperlipidemia [3].

   Systemic bexarotene is approved in the United States for patients with advanced
MF with disease that has been refractory to at least 1 prior systemic therapy.
Bexarotene selectively activates RXRs, as opposed to the RARs. About 80 % of
patients treated with bexarotene develop hypertriglyceridemia, which can result in
pancreatitis if triglyceride levels reach above 800 mg/dL. Another disadvantage of
using bexarotene is that 75 % of patients manifest central hypothyroidism [3]. Mild
increases in transaminases, headaches, skin peeling, and pruritus are among the
disadvantages of using bexarotene [3]. It is important to monitor liver function,
serum lipid levels, thyroid function (serum free T4), and complete blood counts
weekly or biweekly until a plateau in the lipid response, and then at 4- to 8-week
intervals. Lipid-lowering agents and/or thyroid hormone replacement are commonly used to manage these side effects of bexarotene and are usually started prior
to administering the first dose of bexarotene. Importantly, fenofibrate is the preferred agent to control hypertriglyceridemia. Gemfibrozil is actually contraindi-
cated in these patients due to a paradoxical rise in triglycerides when it is combined
with bexarotene.

Interferon

Interferon-α(alpha) (IFN-α[alpha]) is used primarily in the management of relapsed or refractory disease and is the most commonly used biologic response modifier. IFN-α(alpha) can be used alone or in combination with other therapies such as retinoids and phototherapy. When used as monotherapy, it has been shown to result in a complete response rate of 17% and overall response rate of 50% [24].

IFN-α(alpha) has various mechanisms of action that render it useful in the treatment of MF. Tumor cells express a type 1 IFN receptor to which IFN-α(alpha) binds. Upon binding, it can regulate the cell cycle, suppress oncogenes, and modulate cell adhesion. The dosage of IFN-α(alpha) usually starts with 3 MU (million units) per day [25]. Side effects of interferon include flu-like symptoms, leukopenia, elevated transaminases, thrombocytopenia, proteinuria, and myelopathy [11]. It has also been noted to cause depression and confusion [25].

Histone Deacetylase Inhibitors

Histone deacetylase (HDAC) inhibitors represent an emerging drug class for the treatment of MF and have been shown to possess antiproliferative and cytotoxic properties against cutaneous T cell lymphoma (CTCL). Vorinostat and romidepsin have FDA approval for the treatment of CTCL in patients who have progressive, persistent, or recurrent disease following the failure of two systemic therapies. Phase II studies of romidepsin have demonstrated an overall response rate of 34% in MF patients [26]. In another multicenter center study of patients with advanced disease, 26 of 68 patients (38%) achieved a response, including 5 complete responses [27].

Alemtuzumab

Alemtuzumab is an anti-CD52 monoclonal antibody that binds to mature lymphocytes and is used in patients with erythrodermic stage III and IVA, and refractory or progressive stage III and IV disease [18]. It has been associated with an overall response rate of 55%. Adverse events associated with this therapy include serious infections, although lower doses of alemtuzumab administered subcutaneously have shown lower incidence of infectious complications [18]. The NCCN treatment algorithms of stage III and stage IV disease indicate situations in which the use of alemtuzumab can be considered (Figs. 6.4 and 6.5).

Denileukin Diftitox (DAB IL-2)

Denileukin diftitox (DAB IL-2) is a recombinant fusion protein in which the receptor-binding domain of diphtheria toxin has been exchanged for that of the interleukin-2 (IL-2) molecule. The binding of IL-2 to T cells that express IL-2 receptors results in the internalization of diphtheria toxin, leading to inhibition of protein synthesis and resultant cell death of the T cell [11].

DAB IL-2 is a relatively novel therapeutic drug that has shown positive results in stages IB–IVA of MF and refractory MF [11]. Patients are given intravenous DAB IL-2 infusion after premedication with diphenhydramine and corticosteroids. A typical regimen consists of DAB IL-2 infusions for 5 consecutive days, repeated every 3 weeks for up to a total of eight cycles [11]. Adverse events include acute hypersensitivity reactions and vascular leak syndrome, in which patients develop hypoalbuminemia, hypotension, and edema [11].

Chemotherapy

Systemic chemotherapy is typically used in patients with clinically aggressive disease ($\geq$ stage IIB disease or refractory disease) and those with lymph node or visceral involvement. Agents that are used as chemotherapy in MF are similar to those used for other types of non-Hodgkin lymphomas (NHL). Many agents fall under this category; the most commonly used single-agent chemotherapy regimens in MF include methotrexate, liposomal doxorubicin, gemcitabine, low-dose pralatrexate, and purine analogs such as pentostatin (Table 6.1). Other agents that have been used in the setting of single-agent chemotherapy include chlorambucil and etoposide. Temozolomide is considered to be a second-line systemic therapy that has demonstrated clinical activity in NHL and brain cancer, and in the setting of MF, has been shown to have an overall response rate of 33 % in a phase II trial of patients who had already been pretreated [28]. However, further studies are needed to test the efficacy of this drug.

Combination chemotherapy is used for refractory or frequently relapsing disease. A chemotherapy regimen that is commonly used in MF is cyclophosphamide, vincristine, prednisone, and adriamycin (CHOP), which has been associated with partial response rates of up to 90 %, albeit the duration of response may be short-lived [18].

After chemotherapy, interferon-alpha, systemic retinoids, or photopheresis may be used as adjuvants. Systemic chemotherapy is typically reserved for use in the later stages of the disease, as it has not been shown to improve prognosis or overall survival when used in earlier stages [11].

Bone Marrow/Stem Cell Transplantation

Autologous or allogeneic stem cell transplantation, paired with chemotherapy, has demonstrated efficacy in the treatment of late-stage or refractory MF [3]. One of the largest studies of allogeneic stem cell transplant in MF/SS showed that the overall survival rate at 1, 3, 5, and 7 years was 66 %, 53 %, 46 %, and 44 %, respectively [29, 30].

In a series study of 8 patients who had allogeneic transplant, 6 showed no further sign of MF [3]. Recent findings support the use of allogeneic stem cell transplantation in patients who may have failed other therapies and younger patients with refractory MF [31]. Per the NCCN Guidelines, allogeneic transplant can be considered in refractory or progressive disease ≥ stage IIB.

Contributors to This Chapter

- Pooya Khan Mohammad Beigi, MD, University of British Columbia, BC, Canada
- Elizabeth Alice Wang, BS, University of California Davis, Sacramento, CA, USA
- Seyed Sajad Niyyati, BS, University of British Columbia, Vancouver, BC, Canada
- Soneet Dhillon, BS, University of California Davis, Sacramento, CA, USA
- Emanual Maverakis, MD, University of California Davis, Sacramento, CA, USA

References

1. Olsen E, Whittaker S, Kim Y, Duvic M, Prince H, Lessin S, et al. International Society for Cutaneous Lymphomas; United States Cutaneous Lymphoma Consortium; Cutaneous Lymphoma Task Force of the European Organisation for Research and Treatment of Cancer. J Clin Oncol. 2011;29(18):2598–607.
2. Freiman A, Sasseville D. Treatment of mycosis fungoides: overview. J Cutan Med Surg. 2006;10(5):228–33.
3. Galper SL, Smith BD, Wilson LD. Diagnosis and management of mycosis fungoides. Oncology. 2010;24(6):491.
4. Liu DY, Shaath T, Rajpara AN, Hanson C, Fraga G, Fischer R, et al. Safe and efficacious use of intralesional steroids for the treatment of focally resistant mycosis fungoides. J Drugs Dermatol. 2015;14(5):466–71.
5. Van Scott EJ, Kalmanson JD. Complete remissions of mycosis fungoides lymphoma induced by topical nitrogen mustard (HN2). Control of delayed hypersensitivity to HN2 by desensitization and by induction of specific immunologic tolerance. Cancer. 1973;32(1):18–30.
6. Kim YH, Martinez G, Varghese A, Hoppe RT. Topical nitrogen mustard in the management of mycosis fungoides: update of the Stanford experience. Arch Dermatol. 2003;139(2):165–73.
7. Talpur R, Venkatarajan S, Duvic M. Mechlorethamine gel for the topical treatment of stage IA and IB mycosis fungoides-type cutaneous T-cell lymphoma. Expert Rev Clin Pharmacol. 2014;7(5):591–7.
8. Zackheim HS. Topical carmustine (BCNU) for patch/plaque mycosis fungoides. Seminars in dermatology. 1994;13(3):202–6.
9. Zackheim HS, Epstein EH, Crain WR. Topical carmustine (BCNU) for cutaneous t cell lymphoma: a 15-year experience in 143 patients. J Am Acad Dermatol. 1990;22(5):802–10.
10. Zackheim HS. Treatment of patch-stage mycosis fungoides with topical corticosteroids. Dermatol Ther. 2003;16(4):283–7.
11. Gunderson LL, Tepper JE. Clinical radiation oncology. Philadelphia: Elsevier Health Sciences; 2015.
12. Kim EJ, Lin J, Junkins-Hopkins JM, Vittorio CC, Rook AH. Mycosis fungoides and sezary syndrome: an update. Curr Oncol Rep. 2006;8(5):376–86.
13. Heald P, Mehlmauer M, Martin AG, Crowley CA, Yocum RC, Reich SD, et al. Topical bexarotene therapy for patients with refractory or persistent early-stage cutaneous T-cell lymphoma: results of the phase III clinical trial. J Am Acad Dermatol. 2003;49(5):801–15.

14. Breneman D, Duvic M, Kuzel T, Yocum R, Truglia J, Stevens VJ. Phase 1 and 2 trial of bex-arotene gel for skin-directed treatment of patients with cutaneous T-cell lymphoma. Arch Dermatol. 2002;138(3):325–32.
15. Trautinger F. Phototherapy of mycosis fungoides. Photodermatol Photoimmunol Photomed. 2011;27(2):68–74.
16. Herrmann JJ, Roenigk HH, Hurria A, Kuzel TM, Samuelson E, Rademaker AW, et al. Treatment of mycosis fungoides with photochemotherapy (PUVA): long-term follow-up. J Am Acad Dermatol. 1995;33(2):234–42.
17. Rupoli S, Goteri G, Pulini S, Filosa A, Tassetti A, Offidani M, et al. Long-term experience with low-dose interferon-α and PUVA in the management of early mycosis fungoides. Eur J Haematol. 2005;75(2):136–45.
18. National Comprehensive Cancer Network. NCCN clinical practice guidelines in oncology: non-Hodgkin's lymphoma version 3 (2016), Vol. 3 Fort Washington: National Comprehensive Care Network; 2016. p. 105–18.
19. Kim YH, Jensen RA, Watanabe GL, Varghese A, Hoppe RT. Clinical stage IA (limited patch and plaque) mycosis fungoides: a long-term outcome analysis. Arch Dermatol. 1996; 132(11):1309–13.
20. Deeths MJ, Chapman JT, Dellavalle RP, Zeng C, Aeling JL. Treatment of patch and plaque stage mycosis fungoides with imiquimod 5% cream. J Am Acad Dermatol. 2005;52(2):275–80.
21. Martínez-González MC, Verea-Hernando MM, Yebra-Pimentel MT, Del Pozo J, Mazaira M, Fonseca E. Imiquimod in mycosis fungoides. Eur J Dermatol. 2008;18(2):148–52.
22. Duvic M, Martin AG, Kim Y, Olsen E, Wood GS, Crowley CA, et al. Phase 2 and 3 clinical trial of oral bexarotene (targretin capsules) for the treatment of refractory or persistent early-stage cutaneous T-cell lymphoma. Arch Dermatol. 2001;137(5):581–93.
23. Hall JC, Hall BJ. Cutaneous lymphoma: diagnosis and treatment. Shelton: PMPH; 2012.
24. Olsen EA, Bunn PA. Interferon in the treatment of cutaneous T-cell lymphoma. Hematol Oncol Clin North Am. 1995;9(5):1089–107.
25. Spaccarelli N, Rook AH. The use of interferons in the treatment of cutaneous T-cell lymphoma. Dermatol Clin. 2015;33(4):731–45.
26. Piekarz RL, Frye R, Turner M, Wright JJ, Allen SL, Kirschbaum MH, et al. Phase II multi-institutional trial of the histone deacetylase inhibitor romidepsin as monotherapy for patients with cutaneous T-cell lymphoma. J Clin Oncol. 2009;27(32):5410–7.
27. Whittaker SJ, Demierre M-F, Kim EJ, Rook AH, Lerner A, Duvic M, et al. Final results from a multicenter, international, pivotal study of romidepsin in refractory cutaneous T-cell lymphoma. J Clin Oncol. 2010;28(29):4485–91.
28. Tani M, Fina M, Alinari L, Stefoni V, Baccarani M, Zinzani P. Phase II trial of temozolomide in patients with pretreated cutaneous T-cell lymphoma. Haematologica. 2005;90(9):1283–4.
29. Duarte RF, Canals C, Onida F, Gabriel IH, Arranz R, Arcese W, et al. Allogeneic hematopoi-etic cell transplantation for patients with mycosis fungoides and Sézary syndrome: a retrospec-tive analysis of the lymphoma working party of the European Group for Blood and Marrow Transplantation. J Clin Oncol. 2010;28(29):4492–9.
30. Duarte RF, Boumendil A, Onida F, Gabriel I, Arranz R, Arcese W, et al. Long-term outcome of allogeneic hematopoietic cell transplantation for patients with mycosis fungoides and Sézary syndrome: a European society for blood and marrow transplantation lymphoma work-ing party extended analysis. J Clin Oncol. 2014;32(29):3347–8.
31. Mao X, Orchard G, Mitchell TJ, Oyama N, Russell-Jones R, Vermeer MH, et al. A genomic and expression study of AP-1 in primary cutaneous T-cell lymphoma: evidence for dysregu-lated expression of JUNB and JUND in MF and SS. J Cutan Pathol. 2008;35(10):899–910.

Variants of Mycosis Fungoides

7

Clinical and histologic variants of mycosis fungoides (MF) have been reported. Sézary syndrome (SS) is considered to be the leukemic variant of MF and is defined as the triad of erythroderma, generalized lymphadenopathy, and the presence of neoplastic Sézary cells in the blood. In addition to SS, distinct variants of MF include follicular MF, pagetoid reticulosis, and granulomatous slack skin, which each individually have distinctive clinical and histological featured and are classified as separate entities.

Follicular Mycosis Fungoides

Other names of this condition include folliculotropic, follicular, pylotropic, folliculo-centric, and follicular mucinosis [1]. The lesions of folliculotropic MF appear to preferentially affect the face, neck, and upper trunk regions [1]. A highly characteristic finding of follicular MF includes infiltrated plaques in the eyebrow region with alopecia. Histologically, follicular MF is characterized by dense dermal lymphocytic infiltrates localized to the perivascular and periadnexal areas. Folliculotropism is a dominant feature (as opposed to epidermotropism in the case of MF) [2]. The infiltrate contains small- and medium-sized lymphocytes that have irregular and cerebriform nuclei.

Overall survival is poor, with 15-year survival rates of 41 % even in early stage disease [3]. Patients with follicular MF patients are typically less responsive to the standard treatments used for patients with classical MF due to the deep, perifollicular or intrafollicular location of the neoplastic infiltrate [2].

Pagetoid Reticulosis

Pagetoid reticulosis is a T-cell lymphoproliferative disorder and rare variant of MF that was described by Woringer and Kolopp in 1939 [1]. The lesions of pagetoid reticulosis emerge as well-demarcated psoriasiform or hyperkeratotic patches and

© Springer International Publishing AG 2017
P.K.M. Beigi, *Clinician's Guide to Mycosis Fungoides*,
DOI 10.1007/978-3-319-47907-1_7

plaques, often with evidence of central clearing and an elevated, occasionally verrucous, border localized to the extremity [4]. The infiltrates of the lesions are comprised of large atypical pagetoid cells in nests and clusters. Radiotherapy and/or surgical excision are the preferred treatment methods.

Granulomatous Slack Skin

This is a very rare variant of MF. The clinical features of this condition are dark erythematous, atrophic, flaccid, pendular, and redundant cutaneous lesions [1]. These lesions commonly occur in the infolding regions of the skin such as the axillae and groins. Lesions show dense granulomatous dermal infiltrates with atypical T-cells. These infiltrates also contain macrophages and multinucleated giant cells, which destroy elastic tissue [1]. Radiotherapy and/or surgical excision are the preferred treatment methods.

Contributors to This Chapter

- Pooya Khan Mohammad Beigi, MD, University of British Columbia, BC, Canada
- Elizabeth Alice Wang, BS, University of California Davis, Sacramento, CA, USA
- Seyed Sajad Niyyati, BS, University of British Columbia, Vancouver, BC, Canada
- Emanual Maverakis, MD, University of California Davis, Sacramento, CA, USA

References

1. Yamashita T, Abbade LPF, Marques MEA, Marques SA. Mycosis fungoides and sézary syndrome: clinical, histopathological and immunohistochemical review and update. An Bras Dermatol. 2012;87(6):817–30.
2. Kazakov D, Burg G, Kempf W. Clinicopathological spectrum of mycosis fungoides. J Eur Acad Dermatol Venereol. 2004;18(4):397–415.
3. Gerami P, Rosen S, Kuzel T, Boone SL, Guitart J. Folliculotropic mycosis fungoides: an aggressive variant of cutaneous T-cell lymphoma. Arch Dermatol. 2008;144(6):738–46.
4. Harvey NT, Spagnolo DV, Wood BA. 'Could it be mycosis fungoides?': an approach to diagnosing patch stage mycosis fungoides. J Hematopathol. 2015;8(4):209–23.

Part II
Research Study

Background

8

Mycosis Fungoides (MF) and Sézary syndrome (SS) are two common forms of primary cutaneous T-cell lymphomas (CTCLs), which represent a heterogeneous group of non-Hodgkin lymphomas. In MF, an epidermotropic form of CTCL, malignant helper T lymphocytes invade the skin; while patients with SS, a leukemic form of CTCL experience erythroderma and neoplastic T lymphocytes in the blood [1]. MF is a rather rare disease that has an annual incidence of 6 cases per million, which is approximately 4 % of all non-Hodgkin lymphoma cases [2]. MF is observed in all age groups but is most common in older individuals ranging from 55 to 60 years old, with a male-to-female ratio of 2:1. It is also more common in black ethnicities than in Caucasians [3].

MF usually follows an indolent course and an orderly progression from limited to generalized cutaneous symptoms, and noncutaneous or visceral involvement. The cutaneous symptoms are varied and they include patches, plaque, generalized erythroderma, poikiloderma, and itchy skin, as well as papules and tumors [1, 4]. Noncutaneous involvement is uncommon but has been observed in regional lymph nodes, lungs, spleen, liver, gastrointestinal tract, and bone marrow [5, 6]. Diagnosis depends on the type and severity of skin manifestations and noncutaneous involvement [6]. Early diagnosis is difficult when initial patches and plaques are present because of similarities with other skin disorders such as dermatitis or possible mismatch between clinical and pathological findings [7, 8].

The treatment process of MF depends on the stage and biological aggression of the disease, which includes severity of skin manifestations, presence or absence of lymphadenopathy, and severity of visceral involvement. It is believed that only the early stages (IA, IB, IIA) can be fully treated. In these stages, treatment is skin directed and it consists of topical therapies, including steroids and topical chemotherapy agents, such as mechlorethamine and carmustine, radiotherapy, total skin electron beam therapy (TSEBT), and phototherapy [9–13]. On the other hand, direct topical skin treatments may have a number of side effects, such as increased risk of skin cancer due to long-term contact with topical psoralen and ultraviolet A (PUVA) therapy and chemotherapy. In advanced stages of MF, where the disease becomes

© Springer International Publishing AG 2017
P.K.M. Beigi, *Clinician's Guide to Mycosis Fungoides*,
DOI 10.1007/978-3-319-47907-1_8

tumorous (IIB) and erythrodermic (III) and visceral involvement often occurs, no satisfactory response to the aforementioned treatments has been achieved. The aim of treatment in these stages of MF is usually palliation, and various treatment methods are used to improve the patient's quality of life.

Furthermore, clinicians have been looking for alternative, less invasive treatment regimens with the least possible side effects. For instance, interferon (IFN), an immune system regulator, was first tested in 1984 as a treatment for MF patients [14]. It has been shown to have a high rate of response during early stages of the disease [15]. Low doses of interferon-α(alpha) (three million units, three times a week) demonstrated 53 % complete remission (CR) in patients with stage I [15]. Some studies have looked at the possibility of combining PUVA with different doses of systemic interferon therapy in order to reduce the number and doses of PUVA treatments required to make a full recovery [16–18]. Even though at all stages of MF these treatment methods have been proven more effective than interferon monotherapy, their considerable toxicity justifies the search for alternative treatments, such as low-dose interferon, shorter PUVA application, and other maintenance therapies. Unfortunately, there are few studies in the literature that compare PUVA with other therapies or combination treatments. This may be due to the fact that only a few centers have the expertise and experience to deliver electron beam radiation treatment due to its considerable rates of acute and late complications, even though it can produce complete remission [19].

In this section of this book (see Chaps. 10 through 13), I will present the results of our previously unpublished study whose main purpose was to determine and compare the efficacy of two treatment methods, one being PUVA monotherapy and the other being PUVA combined with interferon-alpha-2a in MF patients referred to the Razi Dermatology Hospital in Tehran, Iran. Our efforts focused on the comparison of these two treatment regimens with respect to complete remission, partial remission, different phases of MF, and effect of gender.

Contributors to This Chapter

- Pooya Khan Mohammad Beigi, MD, University of British Columbia, BC, Canada
- Hassan Seirafi, MD, Tehran University of Medical Sciences, Tehran, Iran
- Mohammadreza Ataie, MD, Tehran University of Medical Sciences, Tehran, Iran

References

1. Kuzel T, Roenigk H, Rosen S. Mycosis fungoides and the Sézary syndrome: a review of pathogenesis, diagnosis, and therapy. J Clin Oncol. 1991;9(7):1298–313.
2. Criscione VD, Weinstock MA. Incidence of cutaneous T-cell lymphoma in the United States, 1973-2002. Arch Dermatol. 2007;143(7):854–9.
3. Patel SP, Holtermann OA. Mycosis fungoides: an overview. J Surg Oncol. 1983;22(4):221–7.
4. Kim YH, Hoppe RT. Mycosis fungoides and the Sezary syndrome. Semin Oncol. 1999;26(3): 276–89.

5. Leitch RJ, Rennie IG, Parsons MA. Ocular involvement in mycosis fungoides. Br J Ophthalmol. 1993;77(2):126–7.
6. Weinstock MA, Gardstein B. Twenty-year trends in the reported incidence of mycosis fungoides and associated mortality. Am J Public Health. 1999;89(8):1240–4.
7. Pimpinelli N, Olsen EA, Santucci M, Vonderheid E, Haeffner AC, Stevens S, et al. Defining early mycosis fungoides. J Am Acad Dermatol. 2005;53(6):1053–63.
8. Zackheim HS, McCalmont TH. Mycosis fungoides: the great imitator. J Am Acad Dermatol. 2002;47(6):914–8.
9. Hoppe RT, Abel EA, Deneau DG, Price NM. Mycosis fungoides: management with topical nitrogen mustard. J Clin Oncol. 1987;5(11):1796–803.
10. Ramsay DL, Halperin PS, Zeleniuch-Jacquotte A. Topical mechlorethamine therapy for early stage mycosis fungoides. J Am Acad Dermatol. 1988;19(4):684–91.
11. Vonderheid EC, Tan ET, Kantor AF, Shrager L, Micaily B, Van Scott EJ. Long-term efficacy, curative potential, and carcinogenicity of topical mechlorethamine chemotherapy in cutaneous T cell lymphoma. J Am Acad Dermatol. 1989;20(3):416–28.
12. Herrmann JJ, Roenigk HH, Hurria A, Kuzel TM, Samuelson E, Rademaker AW, et al. Treatment of mycosis fungoides with photochemotherapy (PUVA): long-term follow-up. J Am Acad Dermatol. 1995;33(2):234–42.
13. Gathers RC, Scherschun L, Malick F, Fivenson DP, Lim HW. Narrowband UVB phototherapy for early-stage mycosis fungoides. J Am Acad Dermatol. 2002;47(2):191–7.
14. Bunn PA, Foon KA, Ihde DC, Longo DL, Eddy J, Winkler CF, et al. Recombinant leukocyte a interferon: an active agent in advanced cutaneous T-cell lymphomas. Ann Intern Med. 1984;101(4):484–7.
15. Ross C, Tingsgaard P, Jørgensen H, Vejlsgaard G. Interferon treatment of cutaneous T-cell lymphoma. Eur J Haematol. 1993;51(2):63–72.
16. Roenigk HH, Kuzel TM, Skoutelis AP, Springer E, Yu G, Caro W, et al. Photochemotherapy alone or combined with interferon alpha-2a in the treatment of cutaneous T-cell lymphoma. J Invest Dermatol. 1990;95:198S–205.
17. Mostow EN, Neckel SL, Oberhelman L, Anderson TF, Cooper KD. Complete remissions in psoralen and UV-A (PUVA)-refractory mycosis fungoides-type cutaneous T-cell lymphoma with combined interferon alfa and PUVA. Arch Dermatol. 1993;129(6):747–52.
18. Kuzel TM, Roenigk H, Samuelson E, Herrmann JJ, Hurria A, Rademaker AW, et al. Effectiveness of interferon alfa-2a combined with phototherapy for mycosis fungoides and the Sézary syndrome. J Clin Oncol. 1995;13(1):257–63.
19. Kuten A, Rosenblatt E, Dale J, Leviov M, Tatcher M. Total skin electron irradiation: efficacy in early mycosis fungoides. Leuk Lymphoma. 1993;10(4–5):281–5.

Literature Review

9

Treatment outcomes in 113 patients with mycosis fungoides (MF) and Sézary syndrome (SS) were studied by Anadolu et al. [1]. In their study of 113 patients, 110 were diagnosed with MF while 3 were diagnosed with SS, 101 patients (89.4%) were diagnosed at early phases of the disease (IA, IB, IIA), and 12 (10.6%) were diagnosed at advanced phases (IIB, III, IVA, IVB). The age of diagnosis was between 12 and 81 years (mean 45.6 ± 15.8 years), and 55 patients (48.7%) were male and 58 patients (51.3%) were female. Skin lesion duration varied between 1.5 months and 32 years (average 6.1 years). Psoralen and ultraviolet A (PUVA) was the primary treatment used (91%) at early phases of the disease with a complete remission (CR) rate of 80.4%. Treatment with PUVA + interferon-alpha resulted in 57% complete remission in early phases and 33.3% in advanced phases. Of 113 patients with MF, 8 patients (7% of all patients and 57.1% of advanced phase) passed away, 21.4% of advanced phase patients showed relative recovery, and 14.2% had complete recovery. None of the patients in the early phase died; however, 2 patients (1.9%) progressed to an advanced phase of the disease.

Photochemotherapy in the form of PUVA is the first-line, effective, and tolerable treatment for the early phases of MF. In patients with thin patches and plaques, narrow band ultraviolet B (NB-UVB) is preferred. PUVA is used in patients with thick plaques and those who relapsed after initial treatment with NB-UVB. To induce recovery, three sessions of PUVA treatment per week, or three sessions of NB-UVB per week, were recommended until full recovery of the patient was achieved. In recurrent cases, PUVA monotherapy and/or a combination of PUVA with adjuvants such as methotrexate and interferon were used. Patients in early MF phases showed a good clinical response to combination therapy, such as PUVA with methotrexate, bexarotene, or interferon-α(alpha)-2b. In advanced phases of MF, this combination therapy may be used as first-line therapy. Currently, however, there is no consensus on maintenance therapy using phototherapy in attaining CR [2].

Interferon-alpha-2a was studied as a treatment for T-cell lymphoma in a study conducted by Olsen et al. [3]. In their study, 22 patients with T-cell lymphoma at IA to IVA phases entered into an interferon-alpha-2a controlled study (Roferon-A).

© Springer International Publishing AG 2017

P.K.M. Beigi, *Clinician's Guide to Mycosis Fungoides*,

DOI 10.1007/978-3-319-47907-1_9

Patients received 3 million IU interferon-alpha-2a at first, or received 36 million IU doses as intramuscular injection daily for a period of 10-week induction. At the end of induction, 14 out of 22 patients (64 %) had objective response against tumor: 3 patients had full response, 10 patients had relative response ($\geq$50 % clinical improvement), and 1 patient showed slight response. Responders include individuals who were at IA to IVA phases of T-cell lymphoma and there was at least 4–27.5 months until recovery. Through continued treatment, 3 progressed from partial response to complete response and overall complete response was 27 %. Side effects included acute influenza-like symptoms, which were generally mild and transient. Weakness/fatigue, depression, anorexia, and weight loss were common dose-dependent side effects and were also the most common reasons to decrease the dose. Dose-dependent leukopenia was the most common laboratory side effect seen.

One study performed a systematic review of combination therapy in MF [4]. The results of this study showed that a combination of PUVA with interferon-alpha and/or retinoids does not lead to increased general response. Adding methotrexate but not retinoids to interferon-alpha may increase general response. In MF, no combination therapy is superior to monotherapy [4]. In some cases, patients may benefit from a combination of PUVA with interferon-alpha and/or one retinoid and/or a combination of two latter therapies. In addition, patients at advanced phases of the disease may benefit from a combination of methotrexate and interferon-alpha and/or bexarotene. The combination of bexarotene with vorinostat or gemcitabine does not increase overall response and can in fact lead to more severe complications; thus, it is not a recommended regimen.

The efficacy of interferon-alpha-2a used with phototherapy has been investigated in a study conducted by Kuzel et al. [5]. In their study, 39 patients with all phases of MF and SS were treated with a combination of phototherapy and systemic interferon-alpha-2a. The median follow-up time for the whole group was 28 months. Patients with all disease phases entered the study (IB phase, 14 patients; IIA, 5 patients; IIB, 6 patients; III, 8 patients; IVA, 5 patients; IVB, 1 patient). Overall, 36 of 39 patients showed complete response (62 % CR) and relative response to treatment was observed in 28 %. The response time median was 28 months (ranging from 1 to 64 months). Twenty-nine out of 39 people remained alive, with a median survival time of 62 months (ranging from 1 to 66 months).

Long-term treatment with low-dose interferon-alpha and PUVA in early phases of MF has been investigated in 89 patients with IA and IIA phases [6]. In that study, patients were treated for 14 months with low-dose interferon-alpha-2b (18–6 MU [million units]/week) and PUVA. CR was achieved in 84 % of patients and general response was observed in 98 % of patients. Combination therapy was well tolerated. The most common reason for intolerance to therapy was related to relapse of the disease and not to medication toxicity. Stable recovery was achieved in 20 % of patients.

Rupoli et al. examined treatment with low-dose interferon-alpha-2b and PUVA in early MF [7]. In this study, 25 patients entered the study: 16 men and 9 women between 23 and 80 years. Nineteen patients had phase I MF, and 6 patients had phase II. In the induction phase, the dose of interferon-alpha was titrated to a target dose of 18 MU/week. In the maintenance phase, combination with PUVA led to a reduction in interferon-alpha dose to a maximum of 6 MU/week. After the induction phase, 9 out of 25 patients (36%) showed complete remission (CR) and 15 patients (56%) showed partial recovery (PR). One to 5 months from the maintenance phase, CR was observed in 19 patients (76%) and PR was observed in 5 patients (20%), resulting in an overall response of 96%.

Stadler et al. studied the efficacy of combination interferon-alpha-2a with PUVA photochemotherapy in 16 patients with T-cell lymphoma [8]. Interferon-alpha-2a was administered initially as a subcutaneous injection at a maximum dose of 9 million IU. Simultaneously, photochemotherapy with a maximum dose of 3 J/cm2 was administered. After complete or partial recovery, the interferon dose was continued at 9.3 million IU/week. Photochemotherapy was continued two times per week for at least 2 months and then was ceased according to the phase of the disease. Combination treatment was well tolerated and all patients responded to the initial treatment. Three patients left the study while in the early stages of treatment due to erythroderma after photochemotherapy. Continued photochemotherapy led to complete remission in 10 out of 13 people and partial recovery of 3 patients. After a follow-up period (10–40 months), treatment continued in 4 patients. Treatment in 1 patient due to new Hodgkin disease was ceased.

Ataei and Dadrasmanesh examined a combination chemotherapy method with methotrexate, fluorouracil, and leucovorin in patients with advanced MF [9]. In this study, they evaluated the effects of a new chemotherapy regimen in advanced phases of MF. In this regimen, the synergistic effect of fluorouracil and methotrexate was used. To prevent methotrexate complications, the folic acid derivative leucovorin was used. In this semiempirical study, 5 patients in advanced phases of the disease (IIB phase and above) were selected and placed under multiple sessions of chemotherapy based on the extent to which the disease had been controlled. The results showed that 4 patients had partial response to this method and 1 patient had a complete response. All of them had relapses after increasing treatment intervals. Chemotherapy was well tolerated and no serious side effects were observed. The effects of treatment on tumorous lesions were impressive. They concluded that the therapeutic effects of this chemotherapy approach were not stable, but because of its tolerability and good palliation, this regimen could serve as a viable option for patients.

Contributors to This Chapter

- Pooya Khan Mohammad Beigi, MD, University of British Columbia, BC, Canada
- Hassan Seirafi, MD, Tehran University of Medical Sciences, Tehran, Iran
- Mohammadreza Ataie, MD, Tehran University of Medical Sciences, Tehran, Iran

References

1. Anadolu RY, Birol A, Sanlı H, Erdem C, Türsen Ü. Mycosis fungoides and sezary syndrome: therapeutic approach and outcome in 113 patients. Int J Dermatol. 2005;44(7):559–65.
2. Dogra S, Mahajan R. Phototherapy for mycosis fungoides. Indian J Dermatol Venereol Leprol. 2015;81(2):124.
3. Olsen EA, Rosen ST, Vollmer RT, Variakojis D, Roenigk HH, Diab N, et al. Interferon alfa-2a in the treatment of cutaneous T cell lymphoma. J Am Acad Dermatol. 1989;20(3):395–407.
4. Humme D, Nast A, Erdmann R, Vandersee S, Beyer M. Systematic review of combination therapies for mycosis fungoides. Cancer Treat Rev. 2014;40(8):927–33.
5. Kuzel TM, Roenigk H, Samuelson E, Herrmann JJ, Hurria A, Rademaker AW, et al. Effectiveness of interferon alfa-2a combined with phototherapy for mycosis fungoides and the Sézary syndrome. J Clin Oncol. 1995;13(1):257–63.
6. Rupoli S, Goteri G, Pulini S, Filosa A, Tassetti A, Offidani M, et al. Long-term experience with low-dose interferon-α and PUVA in the management of early mycosis fungoides. Eur J Haematol. 2005;75(2):136–45.
7. Rupoli S, Barulli S, Guiducci B, Offidani M, Mozzicafreddo G, Simonacci M, et al. Low dose interferon-alpha2b combined with PUVA is an effective treatment of early stage mycosis fungoides: results of a multicenter study. Cutaneous-T Cell Lymphoma Multicenter Study Group. Haematologica. 1999;84(9):809–13.
8. Stadler R, Otte H. Combination therapy of cutaneous T cell lymphoma with interferon alpha-2a and photochemotherapy. Skin cancer: basic science, clinical research and treatment. Berlin: Springer; 1995. p. 391–401.
9. Ataei D. Combined chemotherapy of fluorouracil and leucovorin in patients with mycosis fungoides and advanced skin diseases. Journal of Tehran Univerisity of Medical Sciences. 2000;21(5).

Study Goals, Hypothesis, and Design

10

The main purpose of the study presented herein (previously unpublished) was to determine and compare the efficacy of two treatment methods—one being psoralen and ultraviolet A (PUVA) monotherapy and the other being PUVA combined with interferon-alpha-2a in Mycosis Fungoides (MF) patients referred to the Razi Dermatology Hospital in Tehran, Iran. Our efforts focused on the comparison of these two treatment regimens with respect to complete remission, partial remission, different phases of MF, and effect of gender.

Study Goals

The main goal of our study was to investigate the efficacy of two MF treatment methods: PUVA monotherapy and PUVA with alpha interferon (IFN).

Alternative Goals

- Comparison of PUVA monotherapy and PUVA+IFN resulting in complete remission
- Comparison of PUVA monotherapy and PUVA+IFN resulting in partial remission
- Comparison of PUVA monotherapy and PUVA+IFN resulting in an overall response
- Comparison of PUVA monotherapy and PUVA+IFN results as a function of patient's age of diagnosis
- Comparison of PUVA monotherapy and PUVA+IFN results as a function of patient gender

© Springer International Publishing AG 2017

P.K.M. Beigi, *Clinician's Guide to Mycosis Fungoides*,

DOI 10.1007/978-3-319-47907-1_10

Application Goals

Although MF does not have curative treatment, skin-directed therapies, immuno-therapies, and systemic chemotherapies could be applied to induce remission in MF. In our study, two treatment methods that are known to result in complete or partial remission were compared in terms of their efficacy as a long-term treatment option.

Hypotheses to Be Considered

1. The main question is to determine and compare the efficacy of several treatment options
2. Application of cytotoxic methods, by suppression of immune system, could affect treatment results
3. It seems that combination of two treatment methods, PUVA in the form of skin-directed therapy and alpha interferon (systematic immune system boost), can increase the chances of complete remissions
4. Combined treatment methods could result in a truly effective treatment for MF, which could be done through apoptosis of cancer cells, which also boosts the immune system

Design and Method

Study Design

The study is presented as a retrospective study and it included 50 patients diagnosed with MF by the means of biopsy, who were treated with either PUVA monotherapy or PUVA combined with interferon-alpha-2a (IFN-α[alpha]) at the Razi Dermatology Hospital during the years of September 2005 to August 2015. The type and level of skin lesions and presence of lymph node, visceral, or blood involvement according to the Bunn & Lamberg system and then the TNM (tumor, node, metastasis) system were used to determine the stage of MF [1].

Patient information such as age, sex, biopsy diagnosis, stage of MF, location and extent of cutaneous involvement, and type and severity of noncutaneous involvement were collected (Table 10.1). Data collected regarding PUVA monotherapy and PUVA plus IFN-α(alpha) treatment regimens included number of treatments, response to treatment, and adverse effects. After the application of the first treatment, the patients would come in every 2–3 weeks to be reviewed and application of another round of their specified treatment. All patients were followed for a period of 24 months. Furthermore, the treatment responses were then used for comparison, starting with the initial course of treatment (see next chapter).

Table 10.1 Variables investigated in study

Variable	Type of variable		Quantitative quality		Qualitative quality		Scientific definition	Measurement method	Scale
	Independent	Dependent	Continuous	Discrete	Nominal	Ranking			
Age	*			*			Patient's age	Asking the patient	Year
Gender	*				*		Sexual phenotype	Recorded by researcher	Male/female
Disease stage	*					*	Clinical stage of disease according to examination of skin, estimation of involved surface and severity via imaging; lymph nodes and bone marrow biopsy	By specialist	I–IV
Disease duration	*			*			Months passed diagnosis	Chart review/asking patient	Month
Previous treatment	*				*		Previous treatment	Chart review/asking patient	Yes/no
Other diseases	*				*		Any other disease	Chart review/asking patient	Yes/no
Interferon administration	*				*		Under skin administration of alpha interferon during photo therapy	Recorded by researcher	Yes/no
Treatment duration	*				*		Months the patient is being treated	Recorded by researcher	Month

(continued)

Table 10.1 (continued)

Variable	Type of variable		Quantitative quality		Qualitative quality		Scientific definition	Measurement method	Scale
	Independent	Dependent	Continuous	Discrete	Nominal	Ranking			
Accumulated emission dosage	*		*				Total amount of emission received by patient during treatment	Recorded by researcher	Rad
Clinical response level		*			*		Amount of improvement	Recorded by researcher	Entire disappearance of symptoms – 50 % reduction of – No improvement or deteriorate – Increase of lesions size or appearance of new lesions
Side effect		*			*		Appearance of side effects during treatment	Recorded by researcher	Yes/no
Decrease of radiation dosage		*			*		Reduction of radiation due to lesions	Recorded by researcher	Yes/no
Decrease of interferon dosage		*			*		Reducing interferon due to lesions	Recorded by researcher	Yes/no
Stop of treatment		*			*		Stop of treatment due to lesions	Recorded by researcher	Yes/no

Contributors to This Chapter

- Pooya Khan Mohammad Beigi, MD, University of British Columbia, BC, Canada
- Hassan Seirafi, MD, Tehran University of Medical Sciences, Tehran, Iran
- Mohammadreza Ataie, MD, Tehran University of Medical Sciences, Tehran, Iran

Reference

1. Bunn Jr P, Lamberg S. Report of the committee on staging and classification of cutaneous T-cell lymphomas. Cancer Treat Rep. 1979;63(4):725–8.

Treatment Plan

11

The main purpose of the study presented herein (previously unpublished) was to determine and compare the efficacy of two treatment methods—one being psoralen and ultraviolet A (PUVA) monotherapy and the other being PUVA combined with interferon-alpha-2a—in mycosis fungoides (MF) patients referred to the Razi Dermatology Hospital in Tehran, Iran. Our efforts focused on the comparison of these two treatment regimens with respect to complete remission, partial remission, different phases of MF, and effect of gender.

PUVA Monotherapy

Patients were given 8-methoxypsoralen 0.6 mg kg^{-1} PO 2 h prior to UVA exposure. Patients were treated with PUVA three times weekly. Whole body UVA was given in a Dixwell R cabin, which contained 38 UVA fluorescent tubes. Patients wore UVA protective goggles for 24 h after treatment and men wore genital protection. The initial dose was calculated based on Fitzpatrick's skin type (skin type I = 1.5 J cm^{-2}, type II = 2.5 J cm^{-2}, type III = 3.5 J cm^{-2}). The weekly incremental increase was given according to skin type (I = 0.5 J cm^{-2}, type II = 0.5 J cm^{-2}, type III = 1.0 J cm^{-2}). Treatment was based on minimum phototoxic dose (MPD) testing and a 20 % incremental increase was given after each visit, twice weekly. The first eight test doses (0.5, 0.7, 1.0, 1.4, 2.0, 2.8, 3.9, and 5.5 J cm^{-2}) were used for patients with skin types I and II. Patients with skin type III received six doses of 2.0, 2.8, 3.9, 5.5, 7.7, and 10.8 J cm^{-2}.

PUVA Plus Interferon-Alpha-2a

In order to maintain consistency, the patients included in this treatment group were treated with combination of PUVA and low-dose interferon-alpha-2a. For interferon (IFN) treatment, patients received 3 MU of IFN-α(alpha) three times weekly; and

© Springer International Publishing AG 2017
P.K.M. Beigi, *Clinician's Guide to Mycosis Fungoides*,
DOI 10.1007/978-3-319-47907-1_11

for PUVA treatment, 0.6 mg kg^{-1} 8-methoxypsoralen was given 2 h before therapy. The whole body except the genital area was subjected to UVA light treatment three times weekly given through the same Dixwell R machine as the PUVA monotherapy group. It is important to note that patients were given a lower dose of PUVA compared to that of the PUVA monotherapy group. All complete responders received maintenance treatment at the same IFN dose that induced remission until progression of disease or unacceptable toxicity.

Toxicity was scored according to the Common Toxicity Criteria established by the National Cancer Institute [1]. If Grade II toxicity was observed, the IFN-α(alpha) dose was reduced by 25%. If Grade III or higher toxicity was observed, treatment was stopped for 2 weeks before resuming at a reduced dose.

Response Parameters

Response to treatment was considered as complete remission (CR), partial remission (PR), and no response (NR) based on measurements of skin lesions performed at the 2–3 week monitoring intervals:

- Complete remission (CR): complete clearance of all skin lesions.
- Partial remission (PR): >50% reduction of skin lesions.
- No response (NR): any clinical result less than a PR.

Data Analysis

Following data collection, data was entered and analyzed in an SPSS program. The quantitative data was presented as mean and standard deviation; and qualitative data was described through frequency and percentage. Furthermore, Chi-Square test was used to compare the difference between the qualitative variables. Additionally, Kaplan–Meier analyzer and log rank test were also utilized for other statistical analysis, such as comparison of survival rates and remission rates of the treatments.

Data Collection Tools and Method

Clinical examinations, biopsy, immunohistochemistry (IHC), and flow cytometry of peripheral blood and complete blood count (CBC) were done in MF clinic.

Ethical Considerations

There are no specific ethical considerations as both of these methods are reliable and known treatment routines.

Limitation and their reduction methods:

- Patient compliance, including refusal to be referred to MF clinic and phototherapy
- Resource limitations, i.e., costs and accessibility of interferon

Contributors to This Chapter

- Pooya Khan Mohammad Beigi, MD, University of British Columbia, BC, Canada
- Hassan Seirafi, MD, Tehran University of Medical Sciences, Tehran, Iran
- Mohammadreza Ataie, MD, Tehran University of Medical Sciences, Tehran, Iran

Reference

1. Trotti A, Byhardt R, Stetz J, Gwede C, Corn B, Fu K, et al. Common toxicity criteria: version 2.0. An improved reference for grading the acute effects of cancer treatment: impact on radiotherapy. Int J Radiat Oncol Biol Phys. 2000;47(1):13–47.

The main purpose of the study presented herein (previously unpublished) was to determine and compare the efficacy of two treatment methods—one being psoralen and ultraviolet A (PUVA) monotherapy and the other being PUVA combined with interferon (IFN)-alpha-2a—in mycosis fungoides (MF) patients referred to the Razi Dermatology Hospital in Tehran, Iran. Our efforts focused on the comparison of these two treatment regimens with respect to complete remission, partial remission, different phases of MF, and effect of gender.

Study Results

Patient characteristics can be found in Table 12.1. In our study, there were 50 patients with MF, 28 (56%) of which were in the PUVA monotherapy treatment group, and 22 (44%) were in PUVA+IFN-α(alpha) treatment group. The average patient age was 63 years, ranging between 30 and 83 years. In terms of gender distribution, 14 patients (28%) were female and 36 patients (72%) were male as seen in Fig. 12.1. It is important to note that all patients in the IA phase were treated with PUVA monotherapy, but as the disease progressed to later stages, a significantly greater percentage of patients were treated with PUVA+IFN-α(alpha) treatment. As would be expected, a greater percentage of patients in the advanced phases of the disease were placed in the PUVA+IFN treatment group.

As illustrated in Fig. 12.2, 32 patients (64%) were in the early phase of the disease, 14 of which were in stage IA, 14 in stage IB, and 4 in stage IIA; and 18 patients (36%) were in the advanced phase of the disease, 8 of which were in stage IIB, 6 were in stage III, and 4 were in stage IVA. Of these patients, 11 (22%) had no response (NR) to treatment, 13 patients (26%) achieved partial remission (PR), and 26 patients (52%) achieved complete remission (CR). Overall response was calculated among 39 patients to be 78%. In patients with early phases of the disease, 22 of them (68%) achieved CR and 8 people (25%) had PR, and 2 patients (7%) had NR to treatment, so the overall response was 30 patients (93%). In patients with

Table 12.1 Patient
characteristics

Patient characteristics	Number of patients (%)
Gender	
Male	36 (72 %)
Female	14 (28 %)
Age	
Mean	63 years
Range	30–83
Stage of disease	
IA	14 (28 %)
IB	14 (28 %)
IIA	4 (8 %)
IIB	8 (16 %)
III	6 (12 %)
IVA	4 (8 %)
Response to treatment	
No response	11 (22 %)
Partial response	13 (26 %)
Complete response	26 (52 %)

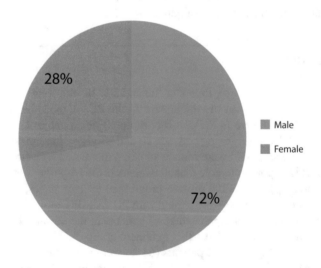

Fig. 12.1 Gender distribution of MF patients

advanced phases of the disease, 4 patients (22 %) achieved CR, 5 patients had PR, and 9 patients (50 %) had NR to treatment, so the overall response was 9 people (50 %). The difference in the response to treatment in terms of early or advanced phases of the disease is statistically significant. In other words, the complete remission and overall response is reduced in advanced phases of the disease, and a greater percentage of patients at advanced phases do not respond to the treatment.

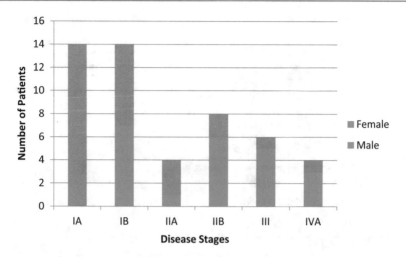

Fig. 12.2 Distribution of disease stages of the MF patients

Table 12.2 A comparison of patient characteristics in both treatment groups

Patient characteristics	Number of PUVA monotherapy patients	Number of PUVA + IFN-α(alpha) patients
Number of patients	28	22
Gender		
Male	20 (71%)	16 (73%)
Female	8 (29%)	6 (27%)
Age		
Mean	65.7 years	59.7 years
Range	30–83	31–79
Stage of disease		
IA	14 (50%)	0
IB	7 (25%)	7 (32%)
IIA	3 (11%)	1 (4%)
IIB	2 (7%)	6 (27%)
III	1 (3.5%)	5 (23%)
IVA	1 (3.5%)	3 (14%)
Response to treatment		
No response	4 (14%)	7 (32%)
Partial response	7 (25%)	6 (27%)
Complete response	17 (61%)	9 (41%)

PUVA monotherapy patient characteristics can be found in Table 12.2 and Fig. 12.3. There were 28 patients in this treatment group: 20 male patients and 8 female patients. The average age in this treatment group was 65.7 years with a range of 30–83 years. In this treatment group, all patients in IA phase (14 patients) achieved the overall response (CR or PR); however, patients in III or IVA phase did

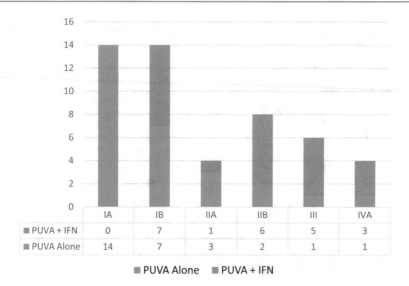

The chart shows the following data:

	IA	IB	IIA	IIB	III	IVA
■ PUVA + IFN	0	7	1	6	5	3
■ PUVA Alone	14	7	3	2	1	1

■ PUVA Alone   ■ PUVA + IFN

Fig. 12.3 Distribution of treatment types of patients with respect to stages of MF

not respond to the treatment. In this group, 17 patients (61%) achieved CR, 7 patients (25%) had PR, and 4 patients (14%) had NR to treatment, so the overall response was 24 patients (86%).

PUVA+IFN-α(alpha) patient characteristics can be found in Table 12.2 and Fig. 12.3. There were 22 patients in this treatment group: 16 male and 6 female. The average age in this treatment group was 59.7 years with a range of 31–79 years. In this treatment group, all patients in IB phase (7 patients) achieved overall response (CR or PR); however, like the PUVA monotherapy treatment group, patients in III or IVA phase did not respond to the treatment. In this group, 9 patients (41%) achieved CR, 6 patients (27%) achieved PR, and 7 patients (32%) had NR to treatment, so the overall response was 15 patients (68%).

Overall, the difference in response to treatment was not statistically significant in comparison between the two treatment groups. In other words, in this study, there was no difference in the response to treatment between the two groups. Moreover, CR was observed in 78.6% of patients in IA phase, 57.1% in IB phase, and 75% in IIA phase. PR was seen in 21.4% of patients in IA phase, 28.6% in IB phase, and 25% in IIA phase. In addition, 66.7% of patients in III phase and 75% of patients in IVA phase did not respond to the treatment ($p = 0.007$). The patient response to PUVA monotherapy treatment can be observed in Table 12.3 and Fig. 12.4, and as seen in the figure all patients in stage IA reached an overall response. Patients in stages III and IVA did not respond to treatment. The patient response to PUVA+IFN treatment can be observed in Table 12.4 as well as Fig. 12.5. All patients in stage IB improved (CR or PR), but similar to the PUVA monotherapy group, patients in stages III and IVA did not respond to treatment. It is important to note that gender

Table 12.3 Patient response to PUVA monotherapy

Response					
Disease type		No response	Partial response	Complete response	Total
IA	Male	0	2	8	10
	Female	0	1	3	4
IB	Male	1	2	2	5
	Female	1	0	1	2
IIA	Male	0	1	1	2
	Female	0	0	1	1
IIB	Male	0	1	1	2
	Female	0	0	0	0
III	Male	1	0	0	1
	Female	0	0	0	0
IVA	Male	1	0	0	1
	Female	0	0	0	0

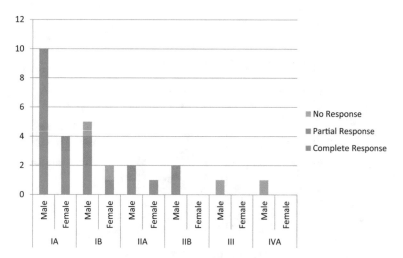

Fig. 12.4 Patient response to PUVA monotherapy with respect to the different disease stages

did not affect treatment response, and there was no significant difference found between the two treatment groups and between various phases of the disease in terms of gender.

Table 12.5 and Fig. 12.6 present relative frequency of treatment response based on disease stage. Complete remission was observed in 78.6 % of IA-stage patients, 57.1 % in IB stage, and 75 % in IIA stage. Furthermore, partial remission was also seen in 21.4 % of patients in IA, 28.6 % in IB, and 25 % in IIA stages; 66.7 % of patients in III stage and 75 % of patients in IVA stage did not respond to treatment ($p=0.007$).

Table 12.4 Patient response to PUVA+IFN

Response		No response	Partial response	Complete response	Total
Disease type					
IA	Male	0	0	0	0
	Female	0	0	0	0
IB	Male	0	1	4	5
	Female	0	1	1	2
IIA	Male	0	0	1	1
	Female	0	0	0	0
IIB	Male	1	2	1	4
	Female	1	1	0	2
III	Male	3	0	1	4
	Female	0	0	1	1
IVA	Male	1	1	0	2
	Female	1	0	0	1

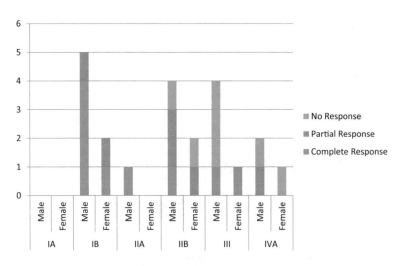

Fig. 12.5 Patient response to PUVA+INF with respect to the different disease stages

Table 12.6 and Fig. 12.7 show the relative frequency of treatment response according to patient sex, and there was no significant difference between the two sexes ($p=0.9$).

Table 12.7 and Fig. 12.8 present the relative frequency of treatment response according to treatment type. There is no significant difference between the two treatment techniques ($p=0.2$).

Table 12.8 shows the relative frequency of complete remission according to type of treatment. There is no significant difference ($p=0.1$).

Table 12.5 Relative frequency of treatment response based on disease stage

Stage of disease	Variables measured	No response	Partial response	Complete response	Total
IA	Frequency	0	11	3	14
	% in this stage	0	78.6	21.4	100
	% of response	0	42.3	23.1	28.0
	Total %	0	22.0	6.0	28.0
IB	Frequency	2	8	4	14
	% in this stage	14.3	57.1	28.6	100.0
	% of response	18.2	30.8	30.8	28.0
	Total %	4.0	16.0	8.0	28.0
IIA	Frequency	0	3	1	4
	% in this stage	0	75.0	25.0	100.0
	% of response	0	11.5	7.7	8.0
	Total %	0	6.0	2.0	8.0
IIB	Frequency	2	2	4	8
	% in this stage	25.0	25.0	50.0	100.0
	% of response	18.2	7.7	30.8	16.0
	Total %	4.0	4.0	8.0	16.0
III	Frequency	4	2	0	6
	% in this stage	66.7	33.3	0.0	100.0
	% of response	36.4	7.7	0.0	12.0
	Total %	8.0	4.0	0.0	12.0
IVA	Frequency	3	0	1	4
	% in this stage	75.0	0.0	25.0	100.0
	% of response	27.3	0.0	7.7	8.0
	Total %	6.0	0.0	2.0	8.0
Total	Frequency	11	26	13	50
	% in this stage	22.0	52.0	26.0	100.0
	% of response	100.0	100.0	100.0	100.0
	Total %	22.0	52.0	26.0	100.0

Table 12.9 shows the relative frequency of overall improvement (CR and PR) according to type of treatment. There is no significant difference between them ($p = 0.1$).

Table 12.10 lists frequency of treatment methods according to the two diseases stages: early and advanced. As it is seen, a higher percentage of patients in advanced stages are in the PUVA + IFN treatment group, which was statistically significant ($p = 0.001$).

Relative frequency of treatment response according to diseases stage is listed in Table 12.11. Most of the patients in the early stages (68.8 %) showed complete remission, while most of the patients in the advanced stages (50 %) did not respond to treatment—a difference that was statistically significant ($p = 0.009$).

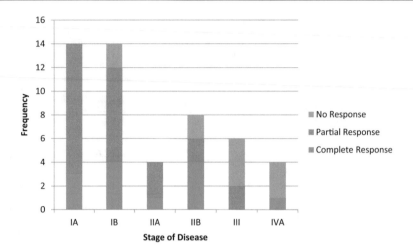

Fig. 12.6 Relative frequency of treatment response based on the different disease stages

Table 12.6 Relative frequency of treatment response based on sex

Treatment response	Variables measured	Male	Female	Total
No response	Frequency	8	3	11
	% in this stage	72.7	27.3	100.0
	% of response	22.2	21.4	22.0
	Total %	16.0	6.0	22.0
Partial response	Frequency	19	7	26
	% in this stage	73.1	26.9	100.0
	% of response	52.8	50.0	52.0
	Total %	38.0	14.0	52.0
Complete response	Frequency	9	4	13
	% in this stage	69.2	30.8	100.0
	% of response	25.0	28.6	26.0
	Total %	18	8.0	26.0
Total	Frequency	36	14	50
	% in this stage	72.0	28.0	100.0
	% of response	100.0	100.0	100.0
	Total %	72.0	28.0	100.0

Table 12.12 shows the relative frequency of complete remission according to disease stages (early or advanced). As shown, 68.8 % of patient in early stages and 22.2 % in advanced stages had complete remission ($p = 0.01$).

Table 12.13 shows the relative frequency of overall remission according to disease stages. As it can be seen, 92.9 % of patient in early stages and 50 % in advanced stages had overall improvement ($p = 0.01$).

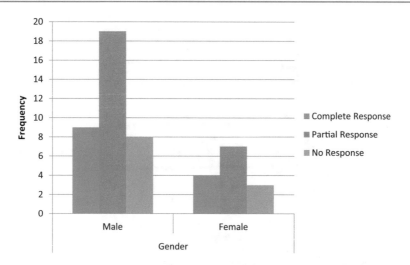

Fig. 12.7 Relative frequency of treatment response based on sex

Table 12.7 Relative frequency of treatment response based on treatment type

Treatment response	Variables measured	No response	Partial response	Complete response	Total
PUVA monotherapy	Frequency	4	17	7	28
	% in this stage	14.3	60.7	25.0	100.0
	% of response	36.4	65.4	53.8	56.0
	Total %	8.0	34.0	14.0	56.0
PUVA+IFN	Frequency	7	9	6	22
	% in this stage	31.8	40.9	27.3	100.0
	% of response	63.6	34.6	46.2	44.0
	Total %	14.0	18.0	12.0	44.0
Total	Frequency	11	26	13	50
	% in this stage	22.0	52.0	26.0	100.0
	% of response	100.0	100.0	100.0	100.0
	Total %	22.0	52.0	26.0	100.0

Figure 12.9 illustrates complete remission in response to treatment type. Using a log rank test, it was determined that the difference in complete remission between the different treatments was not significant ($p=0.2$). In addition, Fig. 12.10 demonstrates complete remission with respect to disease phase, and using log rank test it was determined that the difference in complete remission between different disease phases was significantly different ($p<0.001$). Moreover, Fig. 12.11 illustrates the overall response to treatment with respect to the method of treatment used ($p=0.1$).

Table 12.14 presents the response in the form of complete remission between the two disease stages. There was no significant difference between the treatment groups in the early stages ($p=0.6$) or in the advanced stages ($p=0.8$), which is also shown in Fig. 12.12.

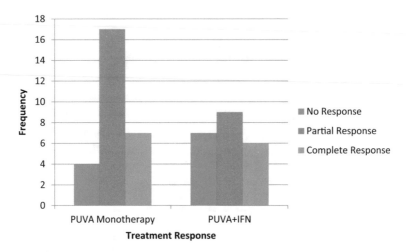

Fig. 12.8 Relative frequency of treatment response based on treatment type

Table 12.8 Relative frequency of complete remission based on treatment type

Treatment response	Variables measured	Complete remission	Incomplete remission	Total
PUVA monotherapy	Frequency	17	11	28
	% in this stage	60.7	39.3	100.0
	% of response	65.4	45.8	56.0
	Total %	34.0	22.0	56.0
PUVA + IFN	Frequency	9	13	22
	% in this stage	40.0	59.1	100.0
	% of response	34.6	54.2	44.0
	Total %	19.0	26.0	44.0
Total	Frequency	26	24	50
	% in this stage	52.0	48.0	100.0
	% of response	100.0	100.0	100.0
	Total %	52.0	48.0	100.0

Table 12.15 shows the response in the form of overall remission (CR + PR) between the two disease stages. There were no significant differences between two treatment groups in the early stages ($p = 1$) or in the advanced stages ($p = 0.4$), which is also shown in Fig. 12.13.

Table 12.9 Relative frequency of overall remission based on treatment type

Treatment response	Variables measured	Overall response	No response	Total
PUVA monotherapy	Frequency	24	4	28
	% in this stage	85.7	14.3	100.0
	% of response	61.5	36.4	56.0
	Total %	48.0	8.0	56.0
PUVA + IFN	Frequency	15	7	22
	% in this stage	68.2	31.8	100.0
	% of response	38.5	63.6	44.0
	Total %	30.0	14.0	44.0
Total	Frequency	39	11	50
	% in this stage	78.0	22.0	100.0
	% of response	100.0	100.0	100.0
	Total %	78.0	22.0	100.0

Table 12.10 Frequency of treatment methods based on disease stage

Treatment response	Variables measured	PUVA monotherapy	PUVA + IFN	Total
Early stages of MF	Frequency	24	8	32
	% in this stage	75.0	25.0	100.0
	% of response	85.7	36.4	64.0
	Total %	48.0	16.0	64.0
Advanced stages of MF	Frequency	4	14	18
	% in this stage	22.2	77.8	100.0
	% of response	14.3	63.6	36.0
	Total %	8.0	28.0	36.0
Total	Frequency	28	22	50
	% in this stage	56.0	44.0	100.0
	% of response	100.0	100.0	100.0
	Total %	56.0	44.0	100.0

Contributors to This Chapter

- Pooya Khan Mohammad Beigi, MD, University of British Columbia, BC, Canada
- Hassan Seirafi, MD, Tehran University of Medical Sciences, Tehran, Iran
- Mohammadreza Ataie, MD, Tehran University of Medical Sciences, Tehran, Iran

Table 12.11 Relative frequency of treatment response based on disease stage

Treatment response	Variables measured	No response	Partial response	Complete response	Total
Early stages of MF	Frequency	2	22	8	32
	% in this stage	6.3	68.8	25.0	100.0
	% of response	18.2	84.6	61.5	64.0
	Total %	4.0	44.0	16.0	64.0
Advanced stages of MF	Frequency	9	4	5	18
	% in this stage	50.0	22.2	27.8	100.0
	% of response	81.8	15.4	38.5	36.0
	Total %	18.0	8.0	10.0	36.0
Total	Frequency	11	26	13	50
	% in this stage	22.0	52.0	26.0	100.0
	% of response	100.0	100.0	100.0	100.0
	Total %	22.0	52.0	26.0	100.0

Table 12.12 Relative frequency of complete remission based on disease stage

Treatment response	Variables measured	Complete remission	Incomplete remission	Total
Early stages of MF	Frequency	22	10	32
	% in this stage	68.8	31.3	100.0
	% of response	84.6	41.7	64.0
	Total %	44.0	20.0	64.0
Advanced stages of MF	Frequency	4	14	18
	% in this stage	22.2	77.8	100.0
	% of response	15.4	58.3	36.0
	Total %	8.0	28.0	36.0
Total	Frequency	26	24	50
	% in this stage	52.0	48.0	100.0
	% of response	100.0	100.0	100.0
	Total %	52.0	48.0	100.0

Table 12.13 Relative frequency of overall remission based on disease stage

Treatment response	Variables measured	Overall response	No response	Total
Early stages of MF	Frequency	30	2	32
	% in this stage	93.8	6.3	100.0
	% of response	76.9	18.2	64.0
	Total %	60.0	4.0	64.0
Advanced stages of MF	Frequency	9	9	18
	% in this stage	50.0	50.0	100.0
	% of response	23.1	81.8	36.0
	Total %	18.0	18.0	36.0
Total	Frequency	39	11	50
	% in this stage	78.0	22.0	100.0
	% of response	100.0	100.0	100.0
	Total %	78.0	22.0	100.0

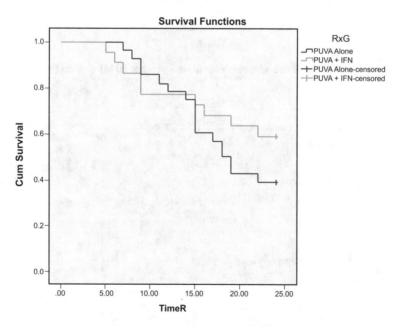

Fig. 12.9 Complete remission in response to treatment types PUVA monotherapy (PUVA alone) and PUVA + IFN of 50 MF patients ($p = 0.2$)

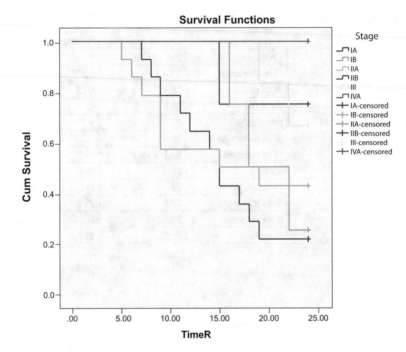

Fig. 12.10 Complete remission with respect to disease phase of 50 MF patients ($p < 0.001$)

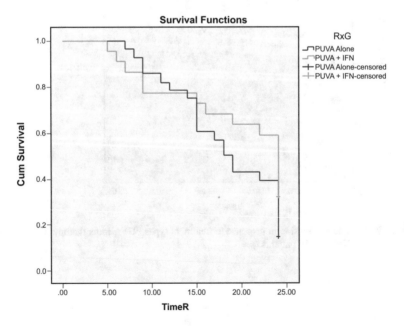

Fig. 12.11 Overall response with respect to disease phase of 50 MF patients ($p = 0.1$)

Table 12.14 Relative frequency of complete remission based on treatment in each stage

	Treatment response	Variables measured	Complete remission	Incomplete remission	Total
Early stages of MF	PUVA monotherapy	Frequency	8	16	24
		% in this treatment	33.3	66.7	100.0
		% of Complete remission	80.0	72.7	75.0
	PUVA + IFN	Frequency	2	6	8
		% in this treatment	25.0	75.0	100.0
		% of Complete remission	20.0	27.3	25.0
Advanced stages of MF	PUVA monotherapy	Frequency	3	1	4
		% in this treatment	75.0	25.0	100.0
		% of Complete remission	21.4	25.0	22.2
	PUVA + IFN	Frequency	11	3	14
		% in this treatment	78.6	21.4	100.0
		% of Complete remission	78.6	75.0	77.8

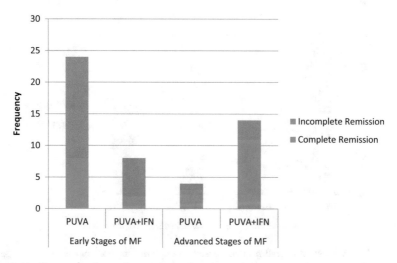

Fig. 12.12 Frequency of complete remission based on treatment method in each of the stages of MF: early ($p = 0.6$) and advanced ($p = 0.8$)

Table 12.15 Relative frequency of complete remission based on treatment in each stage

	Treatment response	Variables measured	Overall response	No response	Total
Early stages of MF	PUVA monotherapy	Frequency	22	2	24
		% in this treatment	91.7	8.3	100.0
		% of Complete remission	73.3	100.0	75.0
	PUVA + IFN	Frequency	8	0	8
		% in this treatment	100.0	0.0	100.0
		% of Complete remission	26.7	0.0	25.0
Advanced stages of MF	PUVA monotherapy	Frequency	2	2	4
		% in this treatment	50.0	50.0	100.0
		% of Complete remission	22.2	22.2	22.2
	PUVA + IFN	Frequency	7	7	14
		% in this treatment	50.0	50.0	100.0
		% of Complete remission	77.8	77.8	77.8

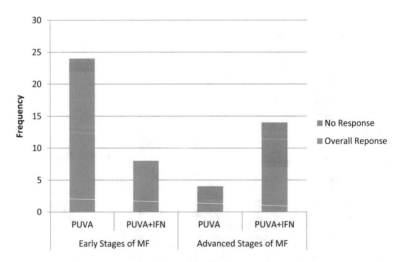

Fig. 12.13 Frequency of overall response based on treatment methods in each of the stages of MF: early ($p=1$) and advanced ($p=0.4$)

Discussion of Study Results

13

Discussion

Treatment of mycosis fungoides (MF) depends on its TNM (tumor, node, metastasis) clinical staging for which psoralen and ultraviolet A (PUVA) has been the accepted standard treatment for early phases of the disease, with reported complete remission (CR) of up to 71.4 % [1]. Researchers have been aiming to find a combination of therapies that will not only work synergistically to result in more patients reaching complete remission but also result in fewer adverse effects, in order to improve quality of life. There are few studies in the literature that compare PUVA with other therapies or combination treatments (see Chap. 9). With that being said, one of the promising treatment combinations reported in the literature has been PUVA plus interferon (IFN)-α(alpha)-2a as it has been shown to require fewer doses of both treatments to reach high overall and complete response rates. For instance, a recent study on the efficacy of PUVA + IFN-α(alpha) reported overall response and complete response of 98 % and 84 %, respectively [2]. In another study done on 89 patients suffering from IA and IIA stages of MF, in which patients were treated for 14 months with a low-dose interferon-alpha-2b (6–18 MU/week) in combination with PUVA, CR was achieved in 84 % of the patients, with an overall response of 98 % [3].

In our own study, there was a significant difference in response to treatment based on the phase of the disease (both in overall and in each individual treatment group). The main purpose of our study was to determine and compare the efficacy of two treatment methods, one being psoralen and ultraviolet A (PUVA) monotherapy and the other being PUVA combined with interferon-alpha-2a in mycosis fungoides patients referred to the Razi Dermatology Hospital in Tehran, Iran. Our efforts focused on the comparison of these two treatment regimens with respect to complete remission, partial remission, different phases of MF, and effect of gender. Of 24 patients in early phase of the disease who were under treatment with PUVA alone, 16 patients (67 %) achieved complete remission, while 8 patients (33 %) did not achieve a complete remission. Among eight patients with early phase of the

© Springer International Publishing AG 2017
P.K.M. Beigi, *Clinician's Guide to Mycosis Fungoides*,
DOI 10.1007/978-3-319-47907-1_13

disease who were under treatment with PUVA + IFN, six patients (75 %) achieved complete remission and two patients (25 %) did not achieve a complete remission. Of four patients who were in advanced phase of the disease and were under treatment with PUVA alone, one patient (25 %) achieved complete remission, and three patients (75 %) did not achieve complete remission. Of 14 patients who were in advanced phases of the disease and were under treatment with PUVA + IFN, 3 patients (22 %) achieved complete remission, and 11 patients (78 %) did not achieve complete remission. Therefore, in examining the response to treatment in terms of complete remission between the two groups separately in subgroups of early phase and advanced phase, a significant statistical difference was not observed.

Of 24 patients in our study who were in early phase of the disease and treated with PUVA alone, 22 patients (92 %) achieved overall response and 2 patients (8 %) did not respond to the treatment. Of eight patients who were in the early phase of the disease and were under treatment with PUVA + IFN, all of the patients (100 %) achieved overall recovery and responded to treatment. Of four patients who were in advanced phase of the disease and were treated with PUVA alone, two patients (50 %) achieved overall response and two patients (50 %) did not respond to treatment. Of 14 patients who were in advanced phase of the disease and were treated with PUVA + IFN, seven patients (50 %) achieved overall response and seven patients (50 %) did not respond to treatment.

After we examined the response to treatment in terms of general remission (complete + partial), there was no statistically significant difference between the two groups in two separate patient subgroups of early phase and advanced phase. Patients in the early phases of the disease responded well to PUVA alone and PUVA + IFN treatment (92 % and 100 %, respectively). In other words, the results of the study showed that PUVA alone and PUVA + IFN are more effective treatments in the early phases of MF. Complete remission and overall response (complete + partial) had no significant difference based on the type of treatment received, using the Kaplan–Meier method and log rank test.

Type and treatment outcome in 113 patients with MF and SS has been investigated by Anadolu et al. [4]. Of 113 patients in the study, 110 patients were diagnosed with MF, and 3 people were diagnosed with SS; 101 patients (89.4 %) were in early phases of the disease (IA, IB, IIA), and 12 patients (10.6 %) were diagnosed with advanced phases (IIB, III, IVA, IVB). Age of diagnosis was between 12 and 81 years (average 45.6 ± 15.8 years). Fifty-five patients (48.7 %) were male and 58 patients (51.3 %) were female. The duration of skin lesion was between 1.5 months and 32 years (average 6.1 years). Psoralen along with UVA (PUVA) was used mostly in early treatment (91 %) phases of the disease and was associated with complete remission (CR) of 80.4 %. Treatment with PUVA + IFN results in a CR of 57 % in early phases and 33.3 % in advanced phases. Of 113 patients with MF, 8 patients (7 % of all patients and 57.1 % of advanced stage cases) died, 21.4 % of patients with advanced stages showed partial remission, and 14.2 % had complete remission. One of the advanced stage patients died, and two patients (1.9 %) progressed to advanced phase of the disease.

In our own study, most patients were in early phases of diseases, with complete remission (CR) measured to be 52 %, and partial remission (PR) 26 %. In our study,

CR was observed in 78.6 % of patients in phase IA, 57.1 % in phase IB, and 75 % in phase IIA. PR was achieved in 21.4 % in IA phase, 28.6 % in IB phase, and 25 % in IIA phase.

Stadler et al. [5] in a randomized clinical trial compared the use of IFN-2a with acitretin and IFN-2a with PUVA in patients with phase I and II cutaneous T-cell lymphoma. In their study, IFN-2a was administered subcutaneously as 9 MU three times a week in both groups. Photochemotherapy was administered after oral dose of 8-methoxypsoralen (0.6 mg/kg body weight) five times a week for the first 4 weeks, three times a week for weeks 5–23, and two times a week for weeks 24–48. For the first week, 25 mg of acitretin was administered daily, and 50 mg was administered for weeks 2–48. Of 98 patients who were randomized in this study, 82 patients were evaluated with phase I and II MF, 40 of whom were in the IFN+PUVA group and 42 of whom were in IFN+acitretin group. Seventy percent complete remission occurred in the IFN+PUVA group. Therefore, this treatment had significant superiority over IFN+acitretin, which had only 38.1 % complete remission. Response time was significantly shorter in IFN+PUVA compared to IFN+acitretin (18.6 compared with 21.8 weeks). Side effects were mostly mild to average, with no significant differences seen between the two treatment groups. However, there were more side effects leading to discontinuation of the medication in IFN+acitretin group.

In Roenigk et al.'s study [6], photochemotherapy either alone or in combination with IFN-alpha-2 in the treatment of cutaneous T-cell lymphoma was studied. In this study, 82 patients with MF and/or parapsoriasis en plaque with PUVA were treated. Clinical and histological parameters were investigated for a period of 6 months to 10 years. Complete clinical clearance of lesions was observed in 51 patients (62 %) and many of them were in the MF group with limited plaques or in parapsoriasis en plaques.

The average total PUVA dose for complete clearance of early MF lesions was lower. Thirty-one patients (38 %) had recurrence and responded to additional PUVA treatment. Patients in early phases of the disease remained in clearance phase for 68 months after the first phase of PUVA. Skin biopsy after treatment in the early phases of MF showed histological clearance. New combination therapy for MF was performed in 15 patients. Intramuscular recombinant interferon-alpha-2a (Roferon-A) along with PUVA was tested. The interferon dose was 6–30 MU three times a week. Disease phases were between I-B and IV-B. Complete response was achieved in 12 patients out of 15 patients, and partial response was in seen in 2 patients out of 15 patients. The overall response was 93 %. Median response time was more than 23 months (ranging from 3 to 25 months). All responding patients were kept on treatment. Symptoms leading to a reduction of dose included fever and weakness (93.3 %), leukopenia (40 %), psychiatric and neurologic changes such as depression and dizziness (33.3 %), and photosensitivity (26.6 %). In conclusion, interferon along with PUVA is very effective regimes for treatment of patients suffering from cutaneous T-cell lymphoma.

In our own study, most patients with early stages of the disease (67.9 %) had complete remission, whereas most patients with advanced stages of the disease (50 %) did not respond to treatment—a difference that was statistically significant.

In a study by Nikolaou et al. [7], PUVA + interferon-α(alpha)2b was investigated in the primary stages of MF resistant to PUVA. In this retrospective study, a combination of PUVA, three times a week and IFN-α(alpha)-2b, 2.5 MU three times a week in 22 individuals was studied. The data of 22 patients were analyzed; seven patients in the early stages of MF were resistant to PUVA, seven were in tumor phase, five patients had erythrodermic MF, and three had Sézary syndrome. The overall response (complete and or partial recovery) was 68 %, including ten cases of complete response (CR) (45 %), and five cases of partial response (PR) (23 %). Significantly more patients from the early phases of the disease, compared to the advanced phase group, achieved CR (86 % versus 27 %, $p=0.03$). In the advanced stage group, CR was 14 % versus 37 % in IIB and III/SS phase patients, but this difference was not statistically significant. Stable recovery (>2 years) was achieved in 5 out of 6 complete responders in the early stage group. The results of Nikolaou et al. are consistent with our own study.

In this regard, in a study conducted by Ahmad et al. [8], 40 patients with MF were treated with PUVA (two times a week) or NB-UVB (three times a week) according to the phase and the extent of the disease. Twelve patients (IIB–IA stages) were treated with NB-UVB and 28 patients (IVA–IA stages) were treated with PUVA. No maintenance therapy was used. In the NB-UVB group, six patients (50 %) achieved complete remission, four patients (33 %) had a partial response, and two patients (16 %) did not show a response to NB-UVB treatment. PUVA resulted in complete remission in 18 patients (64 %), partial remission in six patients (21 %), and lack of response in four patients (14 %). Median time without relapse was 11.5 months in the NB-UVB group and 10 months in the PUVA group. Most patients (79 %) were in early phases of the disease (IA and IB). Of these, 6 out of 10 patients (60 %) in NB-UVB group and 13 out of 21 patients (62 %) in the PUVA showed a complete remission. The results of this study showed that PUVA and NB-UVB are effective treatments in the early phases of MF.

The study of Chiarion-Sileni et al. [9] is a phase 2 clinical trial to evaluate the effect of interferon-alpha-2a with PUVA in patients with cutaneous T-cell lymphoma. In this study, 63 symptomatic patients in all MF and SS phases entered the clinical trial with systemic IFN-alpha-2 with PUVA for 1 year. Then, unlimited maintenance treatment with PUVA was administered to patients who showed complete response. As mentioned, 63 individuals entered the study (IA phase, 6 patients; IB, 37 patients; IIA, 3 patients; IIB, 3 patients; III, 12 patients; IVA, 2 patients). Ten patients had already received treatment. The response time average for the whole group was 37 months. Of 63 patients, 51 patients had complete response (74.6 % CR). Partial response to treatment (PR) was achieved 6 %. The median response time was 32 months. The 5-year survival rate was 91 %, while the 5-year survival rate without disease was 75 %. No life-threatening adverse events were observed. In five patients, IFN-alpha-2a treatment was ceased due to toxicity. Eighty-four percent of patients received more than 75 % of the designated dose (12 million IU three times a week). The study concluded that the combination of IFN-alpha-2a and phototherapy is a safe and effective therapy for patients with MF. The results of their study are consistent with our own study as well.

Conclusion

Patients in the early stages of the disease respond well to both PUVA alone and PUVA + FN treatments. In other words, the results of our study showed that PUVA alone and PUVA + IFN are effective in patients with MF, particularly in the early phases of the disease.

Contributors to This Chapter

- Pooya Khan Mohammad Beigi, MD, University of British Columbia, BC, Canada
- Hassan Seirafi, MD, Tehran University of Medical Sciences, Tehran, Iran
- Mohammadreza Ataie, MD, Tehran University of Medical Sciences, Tehran, Iran

References

1. Oguz O, Engin B, Aydemir E. The influence of psoralen + ultraviolet A treatment on the duration of remission and prognosis in mycosis fungoides. J Eur Acad Dermatol Venereol. 2003;17(4):483–5.
2. Kuzel TM, Roenigk H, Samuelson E, Herrmann JJ, Hurria A, Rademaker AW, et al. Effectiveness of interferon alfa-2a combined with phototherapy for mycosis fungoides and the Sézary syndrome. J Clin Oncol. 1995;13(1):257–63.
3. Rupoli S, Goteri G, Pulini S, Filosa A, Tassetti A, Offidani M, et al. Long-term experience with low-dose interferon-α and PUVA in the management of early mycosis fungoides. Eur J Haematol. 2005;75(2):136–45.
4. Anadolu RY, Birol A, Sanlı H, Erdem C, Türsen Ü. Mycosis fungoides and Sezary syndrome: therapeutic approach and outcome in 113 patients. Int J Dermatol. 2005;44(7):559–65.
5. Stadler R, Otte H-G, Luger T, Henz B, Kühl P, Zwingers T, et al. Prospective randomized multicenter clinical trial on the use of interferon-2a plus acitretin versus interferon-2a plus PUVA in patients with cutaneous T-cell lymphoma stages I and II. Blood. 1998;92(10):3578–81.
6. Roenigk HH, Kuzel TM, Skoutelis AP, Springer E, Yu G, Caro W, et al. Photochemotherapy alone or combined with interferon alpha-2a in the treatment of cutaneous T-cell lymphoma. J Invest Dermatol. 1990;95:198S–205S.
7. Nikolaou V, Siakantaris MP, Vassilakopoulos TP, Papadavid E, Stratigos A, Economidi A, et al. PUVA plus interferon alpha2b in the treatment of advanced or refractory to PUVA early stage mycosis fungoides: a case series. J Eur Acad Dermatol Venereol. 2011;25(3):354–7.
8. Ahmad K, Rogers S, McNicholas PD, Collins P. Narrowband UVB and PUVA in the treatment of mycosis fungoides: a retrospective study. Acta Derm Venereol. 2007;87(5):413–7.
9. Chiarion-Sileni V, Bononi A, Fornasa CV, Soraru M, Alaibac M, Ferrazzi E, et al. Phase II trial of interferon-alpha-2a plus psolaren with ultraviolet light a in patients with cutaneous T-cell lymphoma. Cancer. 2002;95(3):569–75.

Part III

Case Reports

Clinical Research Case Descriptions

14

Case Reports

First Patient

A 29-year-old woman has had lesions for 8 years; the patches were observable on hip, body, stomach, thighs, and forearms. Routine tests were normal, and patches were around 3×4 cm dimension, scaly, without itching. No history of eczema was reported by the patient.

The patient was diagnosed with mycosis fungoides (MF) and treated with narrow band ultraviolet B (NB-UVB) started with 12 s in a total of 89 sessions of phototherapy.

Second Patient

An 11-year-old girl had eczematous spots in her feet, stomach, thighs, back of hips, and back of waist from age 3. She had no itching. The patient was referred with these lesions covering less than 1/5 of the body.

The blood test was normal (i.e., CBC, serum glucose, electrolytes). Also, liver function tests were normal.

She was diagnosed with hypopigmented MF and the patient received 42 sessions of phototherapy (NB-UVB).

Third Patient

A 58-year-old woman with a history of erythematous patches and scaly skin with itching in thighs, underarm, flank, and also severe itching in the hip region. There was no lymphadenopathy appreciated on physical exam.

© Springer International Publishing AG 2017
P.K.M. Beigi, *Clinician's Guide to Mycosis Fungoides*,
DOI 10.1007/978-3-319-47907-1_14

Blood tests were normal, a chest X-ray was normal, and there were no lesions on her head or face.

After diagnosis, treatment was started with Acitretin 25 mg accompanied with UVB. With 20 sessions of phototherapy (NB-UVB), a relative improvement was seen by disappearance of most lesions.

Fourth Patient

An 18-year-old girl presented with MF patches in the right part of her chest, underarm, groin, back of the leg, hip, and back of waist (6 months of disease), without pruritus or lymphadenopathy. She had <10 % body surface area involvement.

Significant improvement was seen after 70 sessions of phototherapy (NB-UVB).

Fifth Patient

A 27-year-old woman presented with MF patches on her forearms, thighs, waist, hips, chest, underarm, and groins. She received 70 sessions of NB-UVB phototherapy. She had no lymphadenopathy on physical exam and no pruritus.

Sixth Patient

A 57-year-old woman presented with brownish patches, 3×4 cm dimension, on her thighs, hips, and hands. She was referred with a 3-year history of lesions.

Diagnosis of MF was made by biopsy from the lesions. After diagnosis, 54 sessions of UVB led to a significant improvement by disappearing of lesions.

Contributors to This Chapter

- Pooya Khan Mohammad Beigi, MD, University of British Columbia, BC, Canada
- Hassan Seirafi, MD, Tehran University of Medical Sciences, Tehran, Iran

Part IV

Clinical Case Photos

Patient One

15

A 45-year-old woman presented with stage 1A mycosis fungoides (less than 10 % of whole body skin involvement), negative HTLV1 serology with mild *pruritus*. After treatment, more than 90 % of lesions healed with phototherapy sessions with narrow-band ultraviolet B (NB-UVB) (Figs. 15.1–15.9).

Contributors to This Chapter

- Pooya Khan Mohammad Beigi, MD, University of British Columbia, BC, Canada
- Hassan Seirafi, MD, Tehran University of Medical Sciences, Tehran, Iran

© Springer International Publishing AG 2017
P.K.M. Beigi, *Clinician's Guide to Mycosis Fungoides*,
DOI 10.1007/978-3-319-47907-1_15

Fig. 15.1 *Patient one*:
Leg lesions before
treatment. Source: Pooya
Khan Mohammad
Beigi, MD

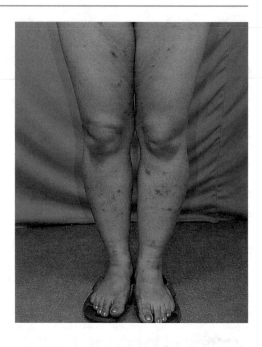

Fig. 15.2 *Patient one*:
Leg lesions after NB-UVB
therapy. Source: Pooya
Khan Mohammad
Beigi, MD

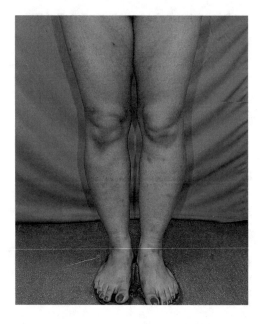

Fig. 15.3 *Patient one*:
Posterior leg lesions prior
to treatment. Source:
Pooya Khan Mohammad
Beigi, MD

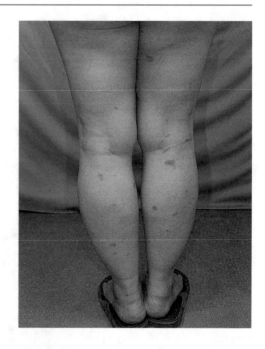

Fig. 15.4 *Patient one*:
Posterior leg lesions after
NB-UVB therapy. Source:
Pooya Khan Mohammad
Beigi, MD

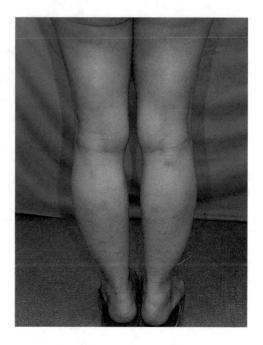

Fig. 15.5 *Patient one*:
Torso lesions prior to
treatment. Source: Pooya
Khan Mohammad
Beigi, MD

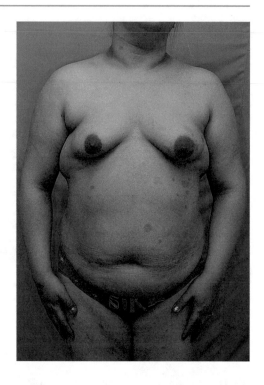

Fig. 15.6 *Patient one*:
Torso lesions prior to
treatment. Source: Pooya
Khan Mohammad
Beigi, MD

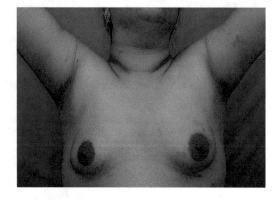

Fig. 15.7 *Patient one*: Torso lesions healed after NB-UVB therapy. Source: Pooya Khan Mohammad Beigi, MD

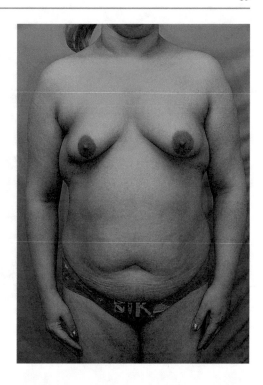

Fig. 15.8 *Patient one*: Posterior view of body prior to treatment. Source: Pooya Khan Mohammad Beigi, MD

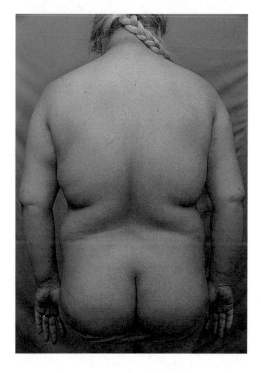

Fig. 15.9 *Patient one*:
Posterior view of body
after NB-UVB therapy.
Source: Pooya Khan
Mohammad Beigi, MD

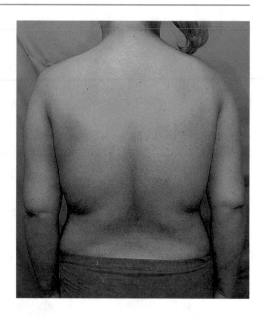

Patient Two

16

A 56-year-old man presents with stage 1B mycosis fungoides (more than 10% of whole skin area involvement), negative HTLV1 serology, and presence of a clonal T cell receptor (TCR) gene rearrangement in polymerase chain reaction (PCR). He was treated with narrow-band ultraviolet B (NB-UVB) and experienced improvement by disappearance of most of his lesions (Figs. 16.1–16.12).

Contributors to This Chapter

- Pooya Khan Mohammad Beigi, MD, University of British Columbia, BC, Canada
- Hassan Seirafi, MD, Tehran University of Medical Sciences, Tehran, Iran

© Springer International Publishing AG 2017
P.K.M. Beigi, *Clinician's Guide to Mycosis Fungoides*,
DOI 10.1007/978-3-319-47907-1_16

Fig. 16.1 *Patient two*:
Torso lesions prior to
treatment. Source: Pooya
Khan Mohammad
Beigi, MD

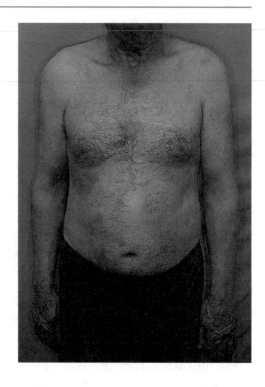

Fig. 16.2 *Patient two*:
Torso lesions healed after
NB-UVB therapy. Source:
Pooya Khan Mohammad
Beigi, MD

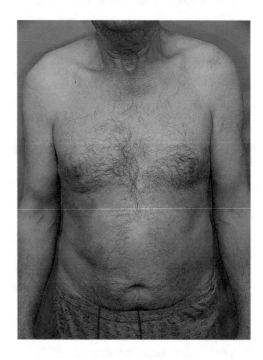

Fig. 16.3 *Patient two*: Posterior view of body prior to treatment. Source: Pooya Khan Mohammad Beigi, MD

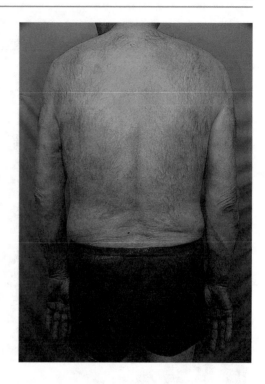

Fig. 16.4 *Patient two*: Posterior view of body after NB-UVB therapy. Source: Pooya Khan Mohammad Beigi, MD

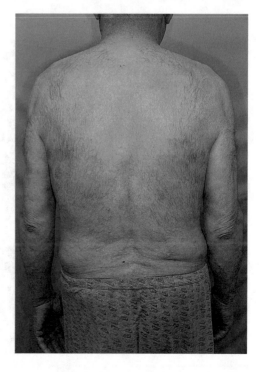

Fig. 16.5 *Patient two*:
Left view of body lesions
prior to treatment. Source:
Pooya Khan Mohammad
Beigi, MD

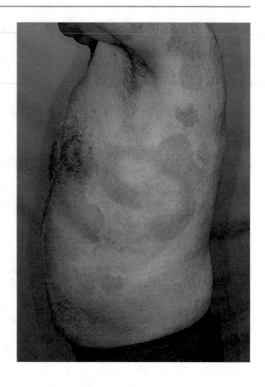

Fig. 16.6 *Patient two*:
Left view of body lesions
healed after treatment with
NB-UVB. Source: Pooya
Khan Mohammad
Beigi, MD

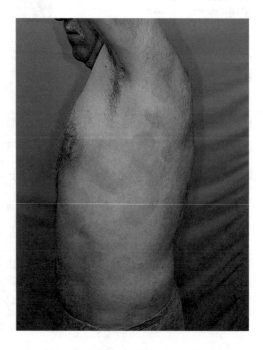

Fig. 16.7 *Patient two*:
Right view of body lesions
prior to treatment. Source:
Pooya Khan Mohammad
Beigi, MD

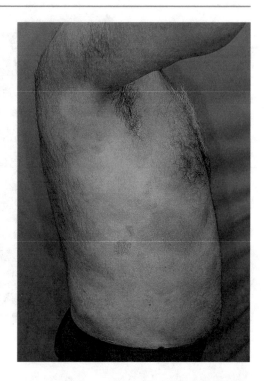

Fig. 16.8 *Patient two*:
Right view of body lesions
healed after NB-UVB
therapy. Source: Pooya
Khan Mohammad
Beigi, MD

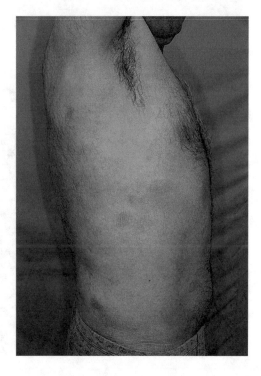

Fig. 16.9 *Patient two*: Front view of legs prior to treatment. Source: Pooya Khan Mohammad Beigi, MD

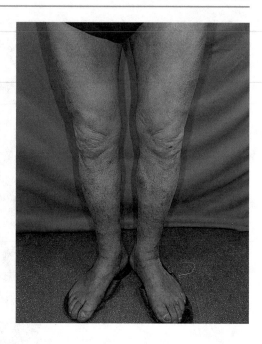

Fig. 16.10 *Patient two*: Front view of legs after NB-UVB therapy. Source: Pooya Khan Mohammad Beigi, MD

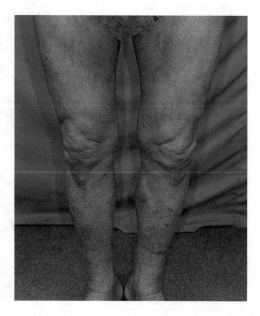

Fig. 16.11 *Patient two*:
Posterior view of legs prior
to treatment. Source:
Pooya Khan Mohammad
Beigi, MD

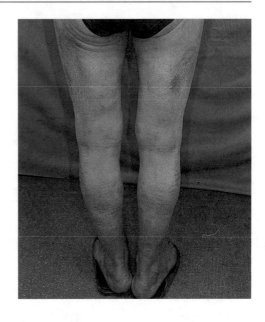

Fig. 16.12 *Patient two*:
Posterior view of legs after
NB-UVB therapy. Source:
Pooya Khan Mohammad
Beigi, MD

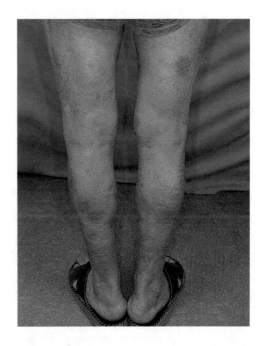

Patient Three

17

A 52-year-old woman presents with reactive axillary lymphadenopathy, negative HTLV1 (Figs. 17.1–17.5).

Contributors to This Chapter

- Pooya Khan Mohammad Beigi, MD, University of British Columbia, BC, Canada
- Hassan Seirafi, MD, Tehran University of Medical Sciences, Tehran, Iran

© Springer International Publishing AG 2017
P.K.M. Beigi, *Clinician's Guide to Mycosis Fungoides*,
DOI 10.1007/978-3-319-47907-1_17

Fig. 17.1 *Patient three*:
Posterior view of body
prior to treatment. Source:
Pooya Khan Mohammad
Beigi, MD

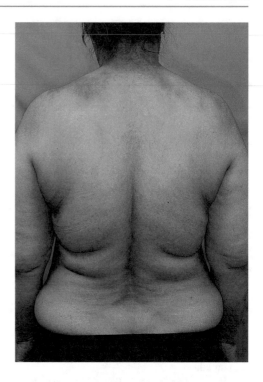

Fig. 17.2 *Patient three*:
Left view of body prior to
treatment. Source: Pooya
Khan Mohammad
Beigi, MD

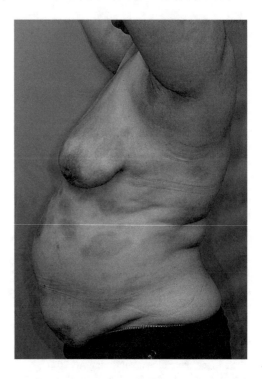

Fig. 17.3 *Patient three*:
Right view of body prior to
treatment. Source: Pooya
Khan Mohammad
Beigi, MD

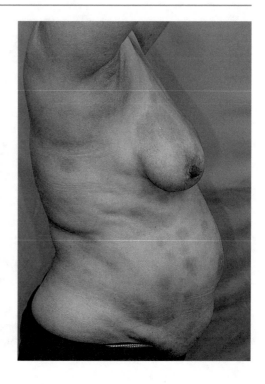

Fig. 17.4 *Patient three*:
Torso lesions prior to
treatment. Source: Pooya
Khan Mohammad
Beigi, MD

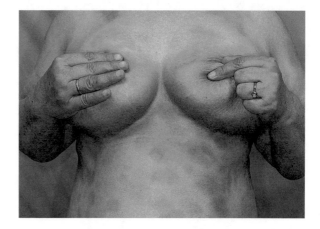

Fig. 17.5 *Patient three*:
Torso lesions prior to
treatment. Source: Pooya
Khan Mohammad
Beigi, MD

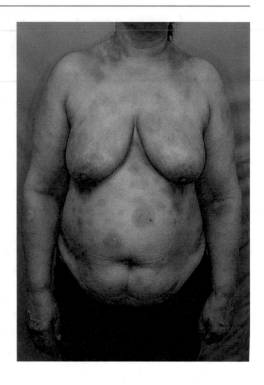

Patient Four

18

A 35-year-old woman presents with stage 1A mycosis fungoides disease (Figs. 18.1, 18.2, 18.3, 18.4, and 18.5).

Contributors to This Chapter

- Pooya Khan Mohammad Beigi, MD, University of British Columbia, BC, Canada
- Hassan Seirafi, MD, Tehran University of Medical Sciences, Tehran, Iran

© Springer International Publishing AG 2017   103
P.K.M. Beigi, *Clinician's Guide to Mycosis Fungoides*,
DOI 10.1007/978-3-319-47907-1_18

Fig. 18.1 *Patient four*:
Leg lesions prior to
treatment. Source: Pooya
Khan Mohammad
Beigi, MD

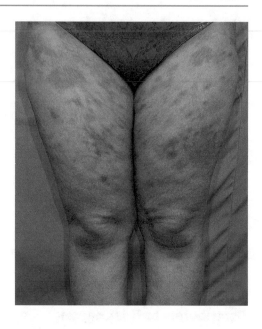

Fig. 18.2 *Patient four*:
Posterior view of legs prior
to treatment. Source:
Pooya Khan Mohammad
Beigi, MD

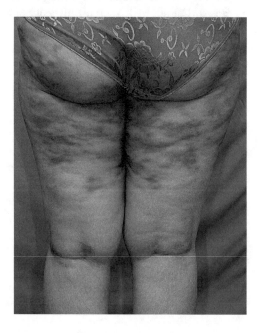

Fig. 18.3 *Patient four*: Posterior view of body prior to treatment. Source: Pooya Khan Mohammad Beigi, MD

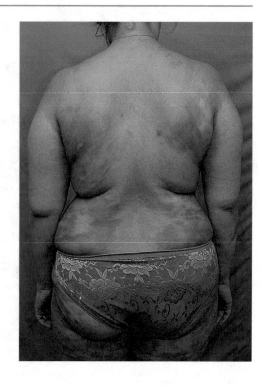

Fig. 18.4 *Patient four*: Axillary and breast lesions prior to treatment. Source: Pooya Khan Mohammad Beigi, MD

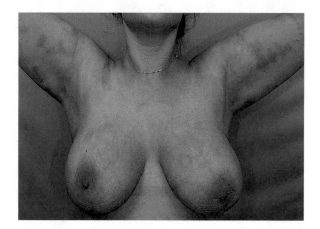

Fig. 18.5 *Patient four*:
Front view of body prior to
treatment. Source: Pooya
Khan Mohammad
Beigi, MD

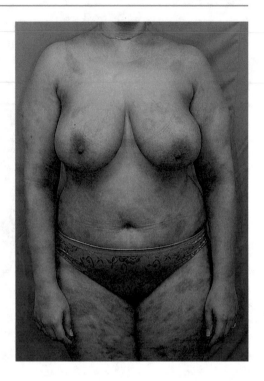

Patient Five

19

A 38-year-old woman presents with stage 1A mycosis fungoides disease, without pruritus, negative HTLV1, and negative T cell receptor (TCR) gene rearrangement with polymerase chain reaction (PCR) (Figs. 19.1, 19.2, and 19.3).

Contributors to This Chapter

- Pooya Khan Mohammad Beigi, MD, University of British Columbia, BC, Canada
- Hassan Seirafi, MD, Tehran University of Medical Sciences, Tehran, Iran

© Springer International Publishing AG 2017   107
P.K.M. Beigi, *Clinician's Guide to Mycosis Fungoides*,
DOI 10.1007/978-3-319-47907-1_19

Fig. 19.1 *Patient five*:
Front view of legs prior to
treatment. Source: Pooya
Khan Mohammad
Beigi, MD

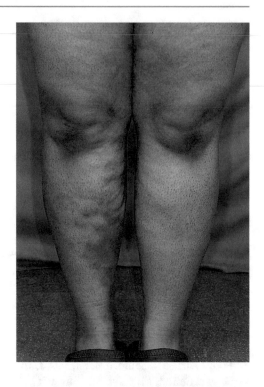

Fig. 19.2 *Patient five*:
Right leg lesions prior to
treatment. Source: Pooya
Khan Mohammad
Beigi, MD

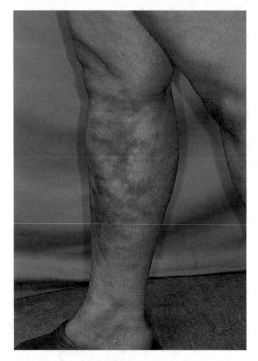

Fig. 19.3 *Patient five*: Posterior leg lesions prior to treatment. Source: Pooya Khan Mohammad Beigi, MD

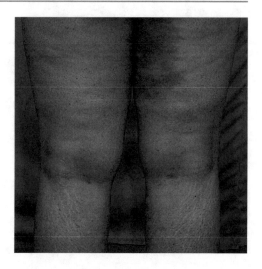

Patient Six

20

A 26-year-old woman presents with stage 1A mycosis fungoides, with negative HTLV1 and negative T cell receptor gene rearrangement with polymerase chain reaction (PCR) (Figs. 20.1, 20.2, 20.3, 20.4, 20.5, 20.6, 20.7, and 20.8).

Contributors to This Chapter

- Pooya Khan Mohammad Beigi, MD, University of British Columbia, BC, Canada
- Hassan Seirafi, MD, Tehran University of Medical Sciences, Tehran, Iran

© Springer International Publishing AG 2017
P.K.M. Beigi, *Clinician's Guide to Mycosis Fungoides*,
DOI 10.1007/978-3-319-47907-1_20

Fig. 20.1 *Patient six*:
Front view of leg prior to
treatment. Source: Pooya
Khan Mohammad
Beigi, MD

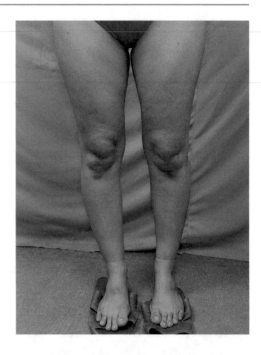

Fig. 20.2 *Patient six*:
Front view of leg after
treatment with psoralen
plus ultraviolet A
phototherapy (PUVA).
Source: Pooya Khan
Mohammad Beigi, MD

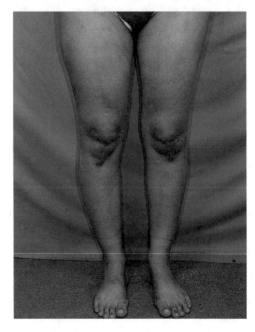

Fig. 20.3 *Patient six*: Posterior view of leg prior to treatment. Source: Pooya Khan Mohammad Beigi, MD

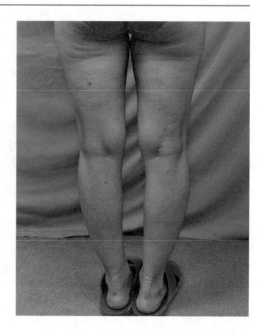

Fig. 20.4 *Patient six*: Posterior view of leg after treatment. Source: Pooya Khan Mohammad Beigi, MD

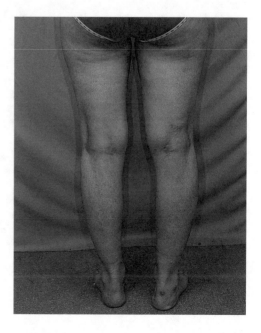

Fig. 20.5 *Patient six*:
Posterior view of torso
prior to treatment. Source:
Pooya Khan Mohammad
Beigi, MD

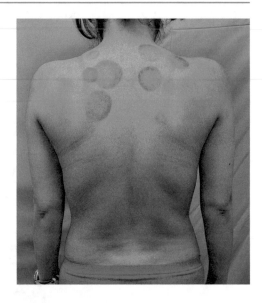

Fig. 20.6 *Patient six*:
Posterior view of torso
after treatment with
PUVA. Source: Pooya
Khan Mohammad
Beigi, MD

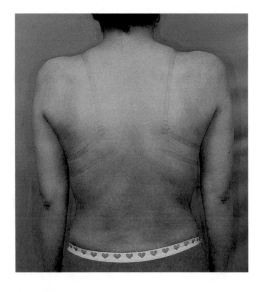

Fig. 20.7 *Patient six*:
Anterior view of torso
prior to treatment. Source:
Pooya Khan Mohammad
Beigi, MD

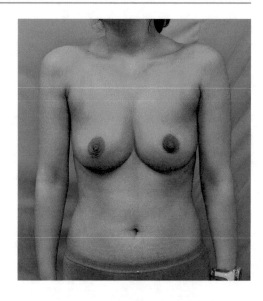

Fig. 20.8 *Patient six*:
Anterior view of torso after
treatment with
PUVA. Source: Pooya
Khan Mohammad Beigi,
MD

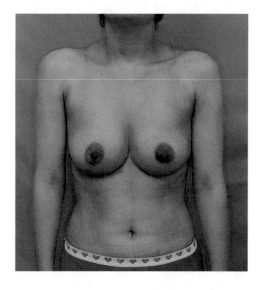

Patient Seven

21

A 27-year-old woman presents with stage 1A mycosis fungoides, less than 5% of the whole body with negative TCR gene rearrangement and negative HTLV1. She achieved complete remission after treatment with psoralen plus ultraviolet A phototherapy (PUVA) (Figs. 21.1, 21.2, 21.3, 21.4, 21.5, 21.6, 21.7, and 21.8).

Contributors to This Chapter

- Pooya Khan Mohammad Beigi, MD, University of British Columbia, BC, Canada
- Hassan Seirafi, MD, Tehran University of Medical Sciences, Tehran, Iran

© Springer International Publishing AG 2017
P.K.M. Beigi, *Clinician's Guide to Mycosis Fungoides*,
DOI 10.1007/978-3-319-47907-1_21

Fig. 21.1 *Patient seven*: Abdominal lesions prior to treatment. Source: Pooya Khan Mohammad Beigi, MD

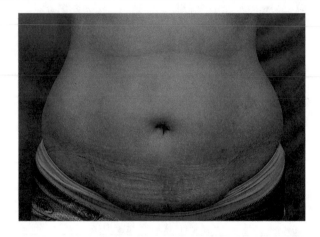

Fig. 21.2 *Patient seven*: Abdominal lesions healed after treatment. Source: Pooya Khan Mohammad Beigi, MD

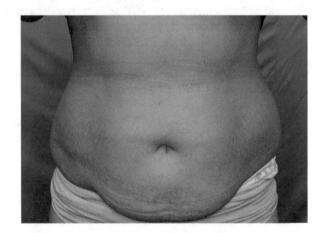

Fig. 21.3 *Patient seven*: Posterior view of hips prior to treatment. Source: Pooya Khan Mohammad Beigi, MD

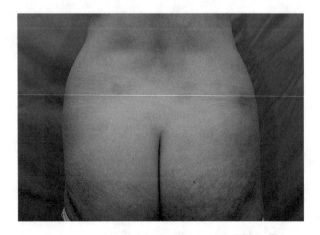

Fig. 21.4 *Patient seven*: Posterior view of hips after treatment. Source: Pooya Khan Mohammad Beigi, MD

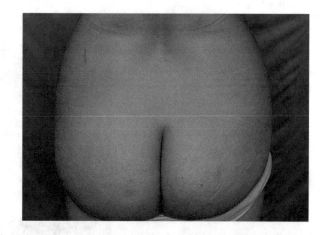

Fig. 21.5 *Patient seven*: Anterior view of legs after treatment. Source: Pooya Khan Mohammad Beigi, MD

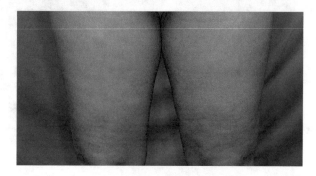

Fig. 21.6 *Patient seven*: Hand lesions prior to treatment. Source: Pooya Khan Mohammad Beigi, MD

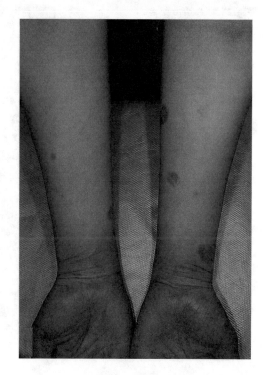

Fig. 21.7 *Patient seven*:
Hand lesions prior to
treatment. Source: Pooya
Khan Mohammad
Beigi, MD

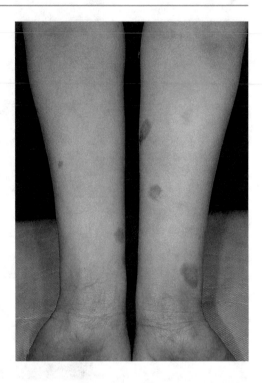

Fig. 21.8 *Patient seven*:
Hand lesions after
treatment. Source: Pooya
Khan Mohammad
Beigi, MD

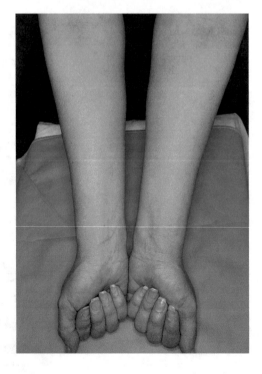

Patient Eight

22

An 18-year-old girl presents with stage 1A mycosis fungoides, with negative TCR gene rearrangement and negative HTLV. She had complete remission of disease after treatment with psoralen plus ultraviolet A phototherapy (PUVA) (Figs. 22.1, 22.2, 22.3, 22.4, 22.5, 22.6, 22.7, and 22.8).

Contributors to This Chapter

- Pooya Khan Mohammad Beigi, MD, University of British Columbia, BC, Canada
- Hassan Seirafi, MD, Tehran University of Medical Sciences, Tehran, Iran

© Springer International Publishing AG 2017
P.K.M. Beigi, *Clinician's Guide to Mycosis Fungoides*,
DOI 10.1007/978-3-319-47907-1_22

Fig. 22.1 *Patient eight*:
Posterior view of legs prior
to treatment. Source:
Pooya Khan Mohammad
Beigi, MD

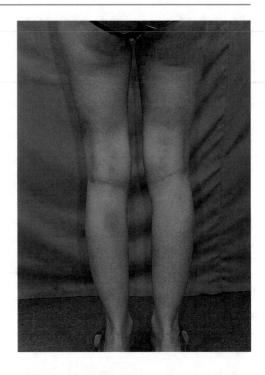

Fig. 22.2 *Patient eight*:
Posterior view of legs after
treatment. Source: Pooya
Khan Mohammad
Beigi, MD

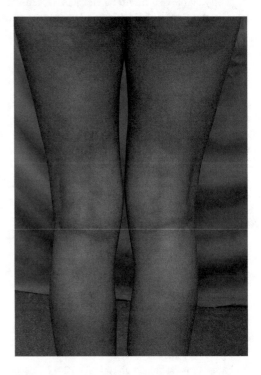

Fig. 22.3 *Patient eight*: Lateral view of leg prior to treatment. Source: Pooya Khan Mohammad Beigi, MD

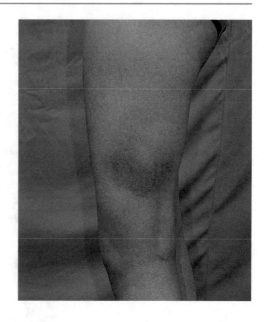

Fig. 22.4 *Patient eight*: Lateral view of leg after treatment. Source: Pooya Khan Mohammad Beigi, MD

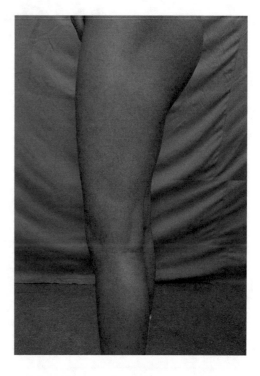

Fig. 22.5 *Patient eight*:
Medial view of left leg
after treatment. Source:
Pooya Khan Mohammad
Beigi, MD

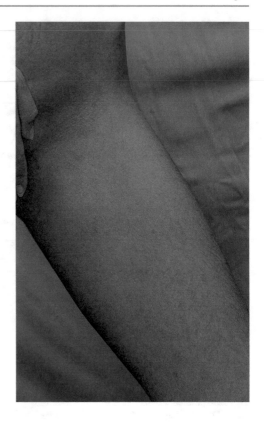

Fig. 22.6 *Patient eight*:
Medial view of right leg
after treatment. Source:
Pooya Khan Mohammad
Beigi, MD

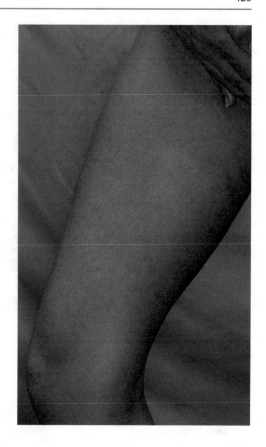

Fig. 22.7 *Patient eight*:
Posterior view of body
prior to treatment. Source:
Pooya Khan Mohammad
Beigi, MD

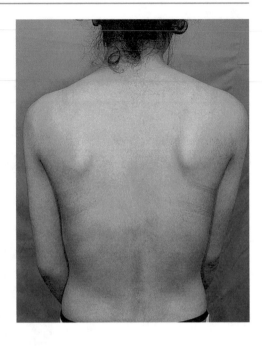

Fig. 22.8 *Patient eight*:
Axillary lesions prior to
treatment. Source: Pooya
Khan Mohammad
Beigi, MD

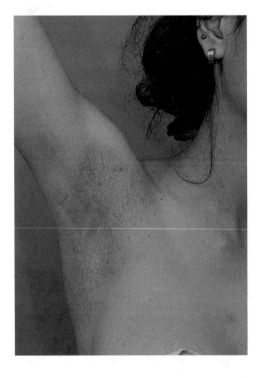

Patient Nine

23

A 54-year-old woman presents with erythrodermic mycosis fungoides, with positive TCR gene rearrangement and negative HTLV1. She achieved complete remission after treatment with psoralen plus ultraviolet A phototherapy (PUVA) (Figs. 23.1, 23.2, 23.3, 23.4, and 23.5).

Contributors to This Chapter

- Pooya Khan Mohammad Beigi, MD, University of British Columbia, BC, Canada
- Hassan Seirafi, MD, Tehran University of Medical Sciences, Tehran, Iran

© Springer International Publishing AG 2017
P.K.M. Beigi, *Clinician's Guide to Mycosis Fungoides*,
DOI 10.1007/978-3-319-47907-1_23

Fig. 23.1 *Patient nine*:
Anterior view of legs prior
to treatment. Source:
Pooya Khan Mohammad
Beigi, MD

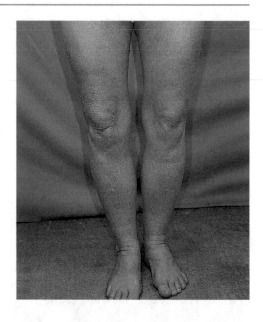

Fig. 23.2 *Patient nine*:
Posterior view of legs prior
to treatment. Source:
Pooya Khan Mohammad
Beigi, MD

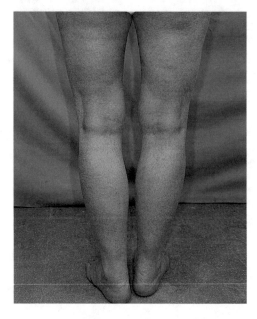

Fig. 23.3 *Patient nine*:
Posterior view of body
prior to treatment. Source:
Pooya Khan Mohammad
Beigi, MD

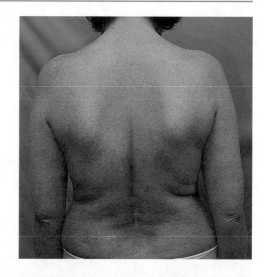

Fig. 23.4 *Patient nine*:
Neck and upper chest
lesions prior to treatment.
Source: Pooya Khan
Mohammad Beigi, MD

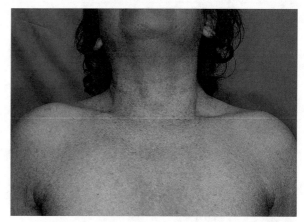

Fig. 23.5 *Patient nine*:
Front view of trunk prior
to treatment. Source:
Pooya Khan Mohammad
Beigi, MD

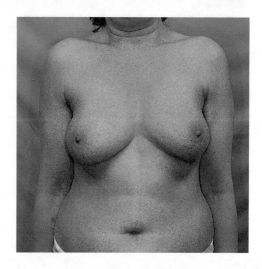

Patient Ten

24

A 42-year-old woman presents with stage 1A mycosis fungoides and negative TCR gene rearrangement (Figs. 24.1, 24.2, 24.3, 24.4, 24.5, 24.6, 24.7, 24.8, 24.9, and 24.10).

Contributors to This Chapter

- Pooya Khan Mohammad Beigi, MD, University of British Columbia, BC, Canada
- Hassan Seirafi, MD, Tehran University of Medical Sciences, Tehran, Iran

© Springer International Publishing AG 2017   131
P.K.M. Beigi, *Clinician's Guide to Mycosis Fungoides*,
DOI 10.1007/978-3-319-47907-1_24

Fig. 24.1 *Patient ten*:
Posterior view of trunk
prior to treatment. Source:
Pooya Khan Mohammad
Beigi, MD

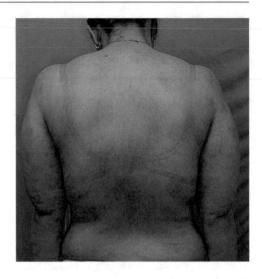

Fig. 24.2 *Patient ten*:
Posterior view of trunk
after treatment with
NB-UVB. Source: Pooya
Khan Mohammad
Beigi, MD

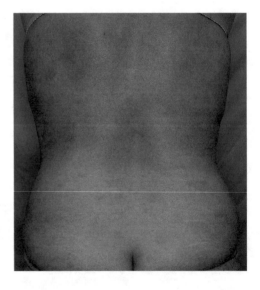

Fig. 24.3 *Patient ten*: Posterior view of legs prior to treatment. Source: Pooya Khan Mohammad Beigi, MD

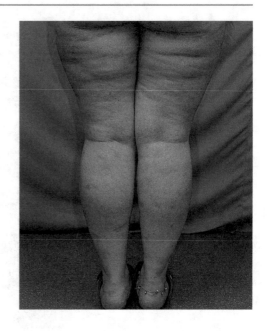

Fig. 24.4 *Patient ten*: Posterior view of legs after treatment. Source: Pooya Khan Mohammad Beigi, MD

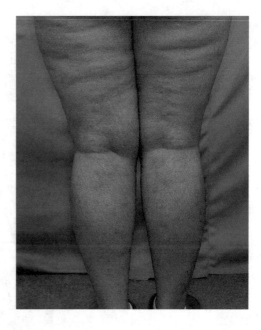

Fig. 24.5 *Patient ten*:
Front view of legs prior to
treatment. Source: Pooya
Khan Mohammad
Beigi, MD

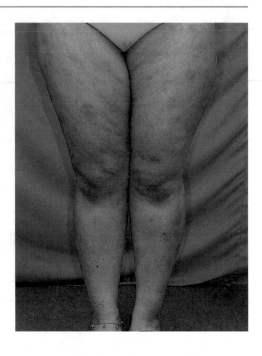

Fig. 24.6 *Patient ten*:
Front view of legs after
treatment. Source: Pooya
Khan Mohammad
Beigi, MD

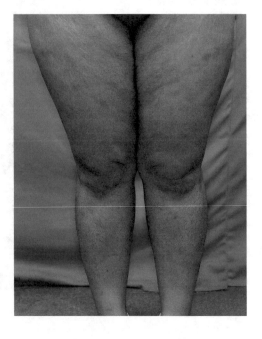

Fig. 24.7 *Patient ten*: Left
arm prior to treatment.
Source: Pooya Khan
Mohammad Beigi, MD

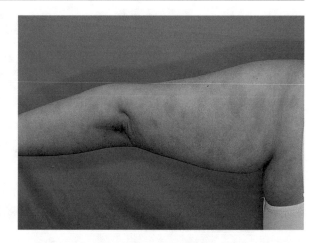

Fig. 24.8 *Patient ten*: Left
arm after treatment.
Source: Pooya Khan
Mohammad Beigi, MD

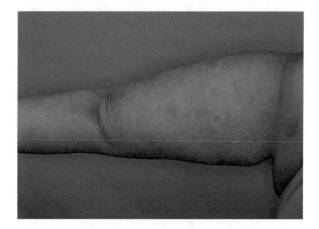

Fig. 24.9 *Patient ten*:
Right arm prior to
treatment. Source: Pooya
Khan Mohammad
Beigi, MD

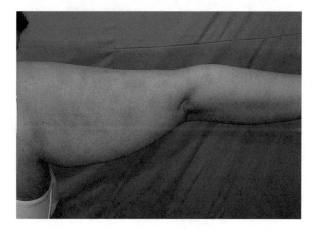

Fig. 24.10 *Patient ten*:
Right arm after treatment.
Source: Pooya Khan
Mohammad Beigi, MD

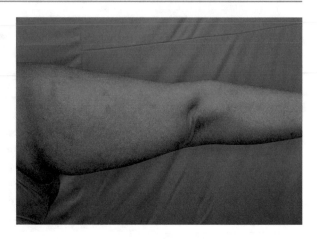

Index

Printed in the United States
By Bookmasters